The Anti-Inflammatory Diet Cookbook for Beginners

Easy Recipes for Chronic Pain Relief and Immune Support

Sophie Nutrify

Introduction

Inflammation is a general biological process. It is part of our immune system's protective response to pathogens or tissue damage. When our body detects an invading pathogen, it discharges immune cells and cytokines to fight against the infection. The process where white blood cells protect the body from infection or injury is generally known as inflammation. It plays a critical role in shielding our body from infection in addition to helping heal injuries. However, when inflammation persists, it becomes destructive and can cause a wide range of health problems, which demonstrates how inflammation is a double-edged sword in our biological machinery.

Inflammation is our body's natural defense system against injury and infections. When our body detects an invading pathogen, the immune response gets triggered. In such circumstances, rather than targeting any foreign invader, our immune system shoots at any target; whether good or bad, any cell or tissue could be made a target. This causes chronic inflammation. In some cases, it attacks our body's cells and tissues, mistaking them for invaders. This process can lead to several chronic diseases, for example heart disease, type-2 diabetes, cancer, arthritis, and many others.

The Misbehaving Immune System problem occurs when the immune response becomes chronic or is activated inappropriately. This may be triggered by many different things, but a major contributor is often lifestyle choices—particularly diet. A bad diet can stir up inflammation, a condition that sets off a cascade of harmful effects that can, among other things, inappropriately activate inflammatory pathways that should remain dormant, setting the stage for many chronic health problems. The most powerful and natural way to reduce inflammation is not by taking drugs, but by eating the right foods. Eating an anti-inflammatory diet focuses on foods that we know are beneficial to the immune system and decrease inflammation. This approach is not about deprivation or cutting things out, but rather about adding in foods that fight disease and support the immune system. This diet is rich in fruits, vegetables, nuts, fish, whole grains, and healthy oils. Specifically, it includes lots of foods that are high in antioxidants and phytochemicals.

Antioxidants are powerful substances that protect the cells in our body from damage. When cells become damaged, they tend to not work as well and may become inflamed. Antioxidants also neutralize free radicals, a group of very unstable molecules in the body that, if left to their own devices, can create massive damage. The proper diet aims to provide the body with nutrients that help the immune system work correctly. The body's immune system must be able to identify malicious threats without dealing harm to healthy cells. Omega-3 fatty acids found in some types of fish reduce levels of inflammatory eicosanoids and cytokines. Meanwhile, dietary fiber found in whole grains benefits certain gut bacteria that play a role in regulating the immune system. Therefore, a good diet should include berries, broccoli, and spices, such as turmeric, which contains antioxidants that suppress NF-kB activation at the cellular level; this molecule plays a key role in initiating inflammation.

Highlighting the anti-inflammatory diet, this cookbook is not just a collection of easy recipes, but also a guide on how to live a healthier life through diet and lifestyle. Every dish is kept simple, so that anyone can follow along and create a healthy dish, regardless of their level of cooking experience. Whether you are looking for a bowl of antioxidant-packed smoothies or a big pot of luscious stew that is also packed with other nutrition, this cookbook has it all. Each recipe starts with preparation and cooking times so that you can plan your time in the kitchen to make sure everything flows smoothly. Additionally, every process of the cooking method is explained so that you won't feel overwhelmed with the finished dish.

Last but not least, nutritional information is included at the end of every recipe, so that you can be aware of the calories, fats, proteins, carbohydrates, and sodium content. This is important for those who count calories and in managing their intake as part of the anti-inflammatory diet. There are many other resources on anti-inflammatory diets, but this cookbook has a unique selling point of not only being user-friendly but also providing scientifically grounded considerations as to how dietary patterns may modulate immune functioning to mitigate the risk of chronic diseases or their manifestations. The aim is not just to share the recipes, but to show that perhaps diet can serve as a mediator between people and their well-being.

When you choose this cookbook, you also choose to step through a door that opens a world where food is not just food, but a means to health and well-being. The meals that you will learn to prepare through this book are like the sweet welcome mat that is laid out for every guest of Planet Health. They are your first steps through the door, taking you from inflammation to rejuvenation.

This cookbook is your guide on this exhilarating journey. It will provide you with the recipes you need to follow the Planet Health program, recipes that you may use for years to come. Here, in this book, we, together, invite you to start enjoying the creative, cleansing, enlivening options that daily meals have the potential to be.

Inflammation is a natural process that the body uses to defend itself against foreign invaders such as bacteria and viruses. It is a protective process that we couldn't live without. In a condition like arthritis, however, the body's defense system or immune system triggers an inflammatory response when one isn't necessary. In other autoimmune diseases, the immune system may target an otherwise healthy part of the body. When this occurs, the immune system—which normally protects the body—causes damage to its tissues. The five major signs and symptoms of inflammation include pain, heat, redness, swelling, and loss of function. Sometimes, only a few symptoms appear, and sometimes, all five are present.

There are two types of inflammation:

- **Acute inflammation:** This is what we call short-term inflammation. You suffer from this when you have a sprained ankle, hurt tissues, or catch a string of bacteria or viruses that need to be eliminated from your body. It can last for minutes or a day if the injury is more severe.
- **Chronic inflammation:** This is a long-term inflammation, during which your immune system starts to attack your body's organs and healthy tissues. Chronic inflammation often lasts for a month or longer, in some cases persisting for years.

Infections leading to chronic inflammation are associated with significant diseases such as arthritis, heart disease, Alzheimer's, cancer, and many more. Symptoms of chronic inflammation, as indicated, are: any autoimmune disorder, insulin resistance, low energy, joint pain, low back pain, skin issues, depression, brain fog, bloating, and poor digestion. Lack of exercise, unhealthy eating habits, continued stressful work, and smoking may be the cause of the infection in the situations mentioned. However, an anti-inflammation diet is an efficient approach to treat the diseases in those situations. It also helps to keep the body weight continuous and save you from the infection above.

Cause of Inflammation

Most of the critical inflammation factors are related to unhealthy eating habits. When we eat a diet high in processed foods, sugars, and unhealthy fats, we constantly cause inflammation. Some of the causes of inflammation are the following:

1. **Daily diet:** Diet is related to one of the most common causes of inflammation. Refined fats and refined carbohydrates are associated with animal products that increase inflammation. According to evidence, red meat, dairy, fried foods, baked food, refined sugar, and highly processed foods saturated with trans fat cause increased inflammation levels in the body.

2. **Infection:** It occurs when harmful agents such as bacteria or a virus enters our body, and our immune system goes into action. It releases cells and proteins to start a process called inflammation, which is similar to getting rid of invading bugs to keep us healthy.

3. **Physical injury:** When we get hurt from something like a cut or scrape, our body reacts with inflammation. This is one of the natural responses produced by our body to protect the injured area and start the healing process. Inflammation is like our body putting up a protective barrier and kick-starting the healing process to recover after an injury.

4. **Foreign bodies:** Foreign bodies such as splinters, dust, and bee stings may provoke inflammation because our immune system will try to crush our outer layer and isolate our organism from the threat.

5. **Chemical irritants:** This includes so-called industrial and environmental irritants. One common and well-studied type of this trigger is irritant contact dermatitis. An environmental irritant damages skin, and the clump becomes bigger, redder, and more irritated. This variant is often seen in the mouth and lungs, too.

6. **Immune reactions:** Immune reactions occur as a result of autoimmune disorders when the immune system mistakes our body's tissues as foreign. These reactions cause chronic inflammation. Chronic autoimmune diseases include rheumatoid arthritis and lupus.

7. **Tissue death situations:** When our body undergoes cell death due to a lack of blood supply—for instance, during a heart attack—or any other kind of injury, our immune system triggers inflammatory cells to clear out dead cells and begin the repair process.

8. **Chronic disease:** Some chronic illnesses cause low levels of inflammation or level states of inflammation that may contribute to disease development. Chronic inflammation may be less apparent than acute inflammation but can be equally severe.

In response to all the causes, the body's immune system initiates inflammation, and the normal process is as I have described. According to this process, the body can repair and protect itself from germs. However, inflammation can manifest differently depending on the cause of the trigger and general health, such as being mild, acute, or chronic. The causes are the key to the management of inflammation due to the various triggers.

The anti-inflammatory diet is a perfect example of a healthy eating lifestyle. You get to eat foods that are densely packed with things your body needs, like antioxidants, macronutrients, micronutrients, and fibers. Since the diet has been designed by a physician, here are some health benefits of an anti-inflammatory diet:

1. **Reduction of inflammation:** An anti-inflammatory diet is one of the healthy diet plans that you can consume even if you don't have inflammation. As mentioned earlier, the foods you eat when you are on an anti-inflammatory diet are rich in vitamins, minerals, fibers, and antioxidants. Antioxidants and resveratrol, which are found in these groups of foods, help to reduce inflammation.
2. **Healthy eating lifestyle:** The diet is appropriate for any person because all the needed amounts of protein, carbohydrates, and fats are present. The diet also encourages eating colorful products: yellow fruits and oranges, tomatoes and berries, dark green leafy vegetables, and cruciferous veggies.
3. **Protect your heart:** The anti-inflammatory diet provides an abundant amount of fiber and healthy monounsaturated fats. There are times when monounsaturated fats are very beneficial because they keep cholesterol levels in check. Also, the anti-inflammatory diet gives you plenty of omega-3 fatty acids, which shield you against heart disease. Your heart will be in top condition if you follow this diet.
4. **Reduce the risk of cancer:** The plant food you consume while on an anti-inflammatory diet is high in antioxidants and fibers as well as contains phytonutrients which help in reducing the risk of cancer. Studies have shown that an anti-inflammatory diet can lower your risk of cancer—prostate, breast, ovarian, lung, and other forms—by helping you maintain a healthy body weight. This also helps in reducing the death count related to cancer.
5. **Improves cognitive function and mental health:** There is a considerable body of evidence pointing to inflammatory processes as mediators behind mental health disorders and cognitive decline. Antioxidants and omega-3 fatty acids are known to have a brain-protective effect against oxidative stress and inflammation. Inflammatory markers have been linked to depression, so an anti-inflammatory diet could have potential benefits in reducing the incidence of mood disorders and age-related cognitive declines such as Alzheimer's, Parkinson's, and more.
6. **Increased energy and better mood:** Many people who follow an anti-inflammatory diet notice increased energy levels and a better mood. This may be due to a decrease in inflammation-related fatigue and a well-rounded intake of vitamins and minerals, which help support hormonal and neurological functions.
7. **Increases lifespan:** Many foods in the diet are loaded with vitamins, minerals, nutrients, fibers, and antioxidants. Antioxidants reduce stomach upsets, oxidative stress, and cell damage. It helps you cut down on inflammatory diseases and increase your lifespan.

Anti-inflammatory food is a great source of nutrients, vitamins, minerals, fibers, and antioxidants, along with their qualities that can build your overall health. They aid in promoting your immune system, cardiovascular health, brain function, and blood sugar levels. Below are some star anti-inflammatory spices, herbs, and ingredients to stock up on, as well as what should be the bedrock of your anti-inflammatory pantry, to keep you feeling and looking healthy while also helping to tackle inflammation.

- **Fresh fruits:** Fruits are one of the good sources of natural vitamins, nutrients, minerals, fiber, and antioxidants. They help to lower inflammation in the body. In this diet phase, consume a large serving of low-glycemic fruits and a moderate serving of high-glycemic fruits.

- **Dark, leafy, green vegetables:** In addition to being chock-full of fiber, dark, leafy, green vegetables also contain inflammation-battling nutrients. Spinach, kale, romaine lettuce, and Swiss chard are great options and include a ton of antioxidants. However, you should also eat vegetables like broccoli, cauliflower, Brussels sprouts, bok choy, and other greens.

- **Whole Grains:** Grains like brown rice, quinoa, and millet are some of the topmost gluten-free foods for inflammation. Aim to consume whole grains three to five times a day to get optimal results. When purchasing gluten-free whole grains, always make sure to look for the gluten-free label on the product.

- **Healthy fats:** They are also a good source of energy and healthy fats. They will give you 30%–40% fat energy while you are on an anti-inflammatory diet. It helps to maintain your cholesterol levels as well as regulate your blood sugar level and input of appetite. It also keeps you full for a long time.

- **Herbs and spices:** These do not only make you inflammation-free, but also enhance flavor. For instance, turmeric, peppermint, thyme, black pepper, ginger, cloves, rosemary, sage, cinnamon, and garlic in an anti-inflammatory diet helps to reduce inflammation in the body.

- **Seafood:** Seafood is one of the great sources of protein and omega-3 fatty acids. Omega-3 fatty acids are good for maintaining heart health, hormones, brain function, etc. Seafood is also important for reducing inflammation. Healthy examples of seafood include fatty fish like tuna, albacore, salmon, lake trout, sardines, mackerel, lean fish, shellfish, other cold-water fish, shrimp, mackerel, and cod.

- **Probiotics:** Probiotics refer to nothing other than healthy bacteria, including lactobacilli and bifid bacteria. In some ways, the probiotics are anti-inflammatory, especially, in constipation treatment, diarrhea, and inflammatory diseases. Products derived from fermented dairy, including yogurt, kefir, and soy-based beverages, contribute to the increase of probiotic bacteria.

Starting a healthy diet isn't always easy, but it can be one of the most powerful actions you ever take to become healthier. Here are my top ten practical steps to support you in successfully embracing an anti-inflammatory way of eating:

1. **Choose whole foods**
   Consume natural, whole foods, such as fruits, vegetables, whole grains, and lean proteins. Avoid processed foods that contain ingredients such as sugar and white flour which can aggravate inflammation.

2. **Incorporate anti-inflammatory fats**
   Use olive oil, avocado, and nuts to replace saturated and trans fats, as monounsaturated and omega-3 fats are anti-inflammatory.

3. **Eat a variety of fruits and veggies**
   Fill half your dish with fruits and veggies in rainbow hues at each feast; they're excellent sources of anti-inflammatory antioxidants and phytochemicals.

4. **Choose whole grains over refined**
   Buck the white pasta and choose brown rice, quinoa, and cricket flour-based whole-wheat pasta instead. Whole forms offer all the nutrition, and the fibers help in curtailing the inflammation process.

5. **Include omega-3-rich food in your diet**
   Seafood like salmon and mackerel, and nuts like flaxseeds and walnuts are omega-3 fatty acid-rich foods. This nutrient has anti-inflammatory properties. So, it is beneficial to consume them multiple days per week.

6. **Season the food with herbs and spices**
   Turmeric, ginger, basil, clove—amino acids have powerful anti-inflammatory agents. Thus, add them generously when cooking.

7. **Limit added sugars and salt**
   Sugar and salt consumed in excess can cause inflammation. Stay away from sugary drinks and snacks and packaged processed foods, as these often contain significant amounts of both.

8. **Stay hydrated**
   Hydration is an important factor in cellular health and inflammation reduction. Drink enough water each day—at least 8 glasses, or more if you live in a hot climate.

9. **Plan for your meals**
   Meal prepping each week can help you to inculcate a variety of anti-inflammatory foods, reducing the likelihood of opting for a less healthy choice when you are undecided about what to eat.

10. Be patient and keep going

Transitioning to an anti-inflammatory diet is not something that is going to happen overnight. You should be patient and make gradual changes to your diet instead of trying to change overnight. You also need to be persistent and stick with it to realize the full benefits of this healthy and nutritious eating behavior.

Chapter 2—Breakfast Recipes

1-Turmeric Oatmeal

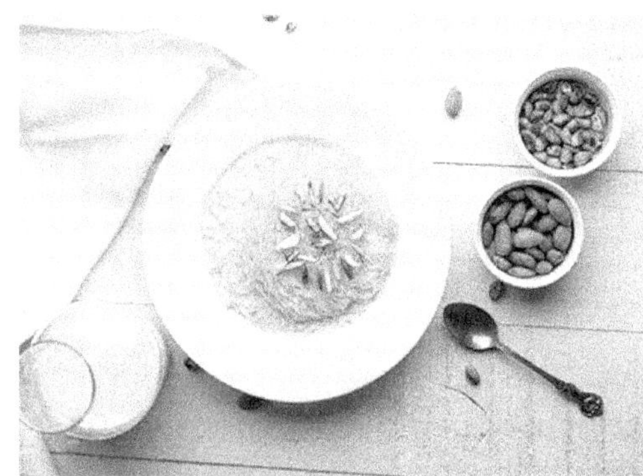

Preparation Time: 5 minutes
Cooking Time: 5 minutes
Serves: 2
Ingredients:

- 1 cup rolled oats
- ½ tsp ground ginger
- 1 tsp ground cinnamon
- 1 tsp turmeric
- 2 tsp maple syrup
- 2 tbsp ground flaxseed
- 2 cups unsweetened almond milk
- Salt

Directions:

Add oats and remaining ingredients in a small saucepan, stir well, and cook over medium-low heat.

Turn heat to low and simmer for 4–5 minutes or until oats become fluffy.

Serve immediately and enjoy.

Nutritional Data: 317 calories | 63.38g carbs | 10.73g fat | 11.77g protein | 177mg sodium

2- Chia Seed Pudding

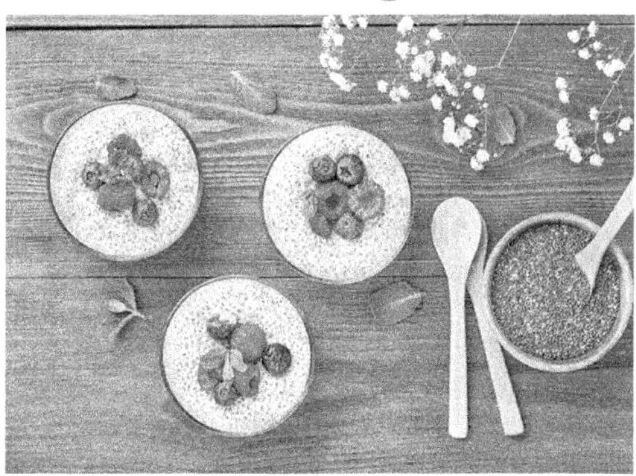

Preparation Time: 5 minutes
Cooking Time: 5 minutes
Serves: 4
Ingredients:

- ½ cup chia seeds
- ½ tsp ground ginger
- ½ tsp ground cinnamon
- 1 tsp ground turmeric
- 1 tsp vanilla
- 3 tbsp honey
- 4 cups coconut milk

Directions:

In a mixing bowl, mix coconut milk, honey, vanilla, turmeric, cinnamon and ginger. Add chia seeds, mix well, and set aside for 5 minutes.

Cover bowl and place in refrigerator for 8 hours.

Divide pudding into four serving glasses and top with fresh berries.

Serve and enjoy.

Nutritional Data: 704 calories | 35.76g carbs | 63.4g fat | 8.96g protein | 40mg sodium

3- Avocado Toast

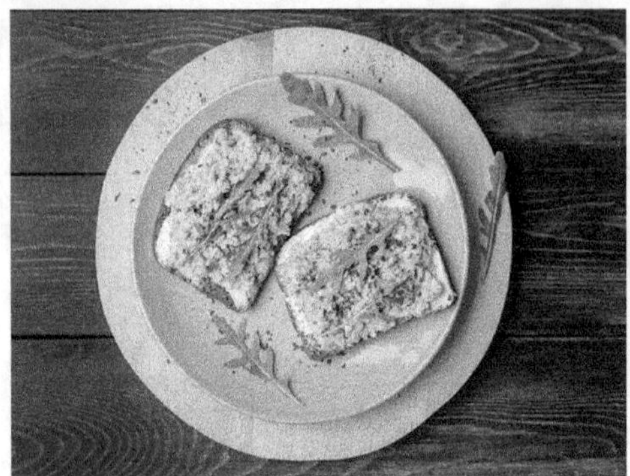

Preparation Time: 5 minutes
Cooking Time: 5 minutes
Serves: 1
Ingredients:

- ½ avocado, flesh scooped out
- 1 whole-grain bread slice
- 1 tsp olive oil
- 1 tsp fresh lemon juice
- ½ tsp red pepper flakes
- Pepper
- Salt

Directions:

Toast bread slices in a pan over medium heat with olive oil.

Add avocado flesh in a small bowl and mash using a fork. Add lemon juice, red pepper flakes, pepper, and salt and mix until well combined.

Spread the avocado mixture on top of the toasted bread slice evenly.

Serve and enjoy.

Nutritional Data: 337 calories | 33.08g carbs | 21.11g fat | 8.86g protein | 168mg sodium

4- Smoothie Bowl

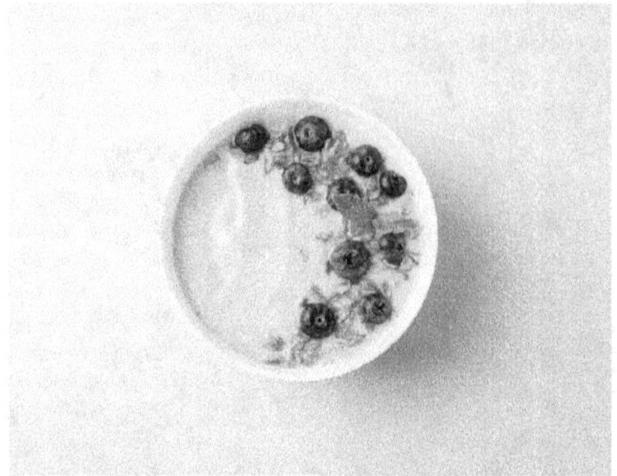

Preparation Time: 5 minutes
Cooking Time: 5 minutes
Serves: 2
Ingredients:

- 1/4 cup Greek yogurt
- 2 tbsp granola
- 2 tbsp pumpkin seeds
- 1 cup fresh strawberries
- 1 cup blueberries
- 1/4 cup blackberries
- 1 cup fresh raspberries
- 1 frozen banana
- 1 tbsp flaxseeds
- 1/2 cup crushed ice

Directions:

Add banana, blueberries, raspberries, strawberries, yogurt, and crushed ice in a blender and blend until smooth.

Divide the smoothie between two serving bowls and top each with granola, flaxseeds, pumpkin seeds, and blackberries.

Serve and enjoy.

Nutritional Data: 495 calories | 95.62g carbs | 11.15g fat | 10.95g protein | 58mg sodium

5-Sweet Potato Hash

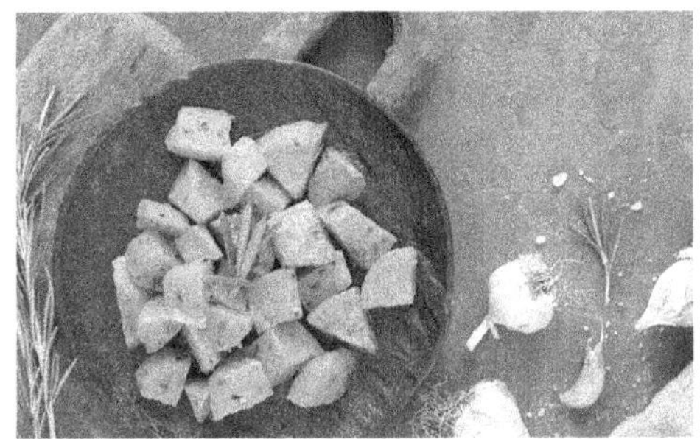

Preparation Time: 10 minutes
Cooking Time: 65 minutes
Serves: 6
Ingredients:

- 6 cups sweet potatoes, peeled and diced
- 1 onion, diced
- 6 garlic cloves, minced
- 1/3 cup olive oil
- 1/2 tsp paprika
- 1/2 tsp pepper
- 1 tsp thyme
- 1 tsp onion powder
- 1 tbsp garlic powder
- 2 tsp salt

Directions:

Preheat oven to 450°F.

Add sweet potatoes to a casserole dish and sprinkle with paprika, thyme, garlic powder, pepper, onion powder, and salt.

Drizzle oil over sweet potatoes and toss well.

Roast in preheated oven for 55–65 minutes. Stir 3–4 times.

Heat 1 tablespoon of olive oil in a pan over medium heat.

Add onion and garlic and sauté for 12–15 minutes.

Once sweet potatoes are cooked, remove from oven.

Add onion and garlic mixture to the sweet potatoes and stir well.

Serve and enjoy.

Nutritional Data: 140 calories | 7.78g carbs | 12.15g fat | 1.68g protein | 780mg sodium

6- Quinoa Breakfast Bowl

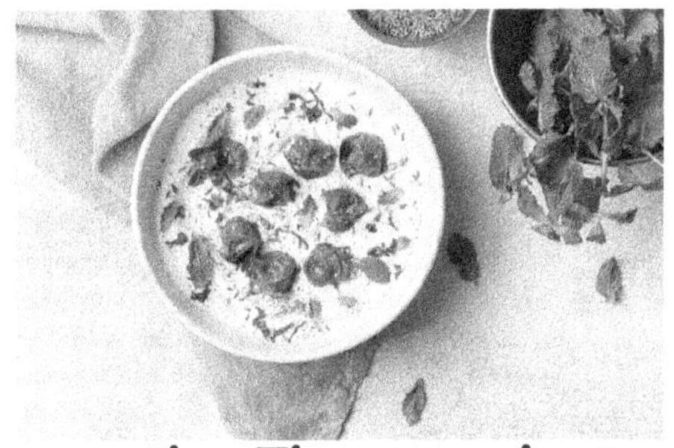

Preparation Time: 10 minutes
Cooking Time: 20 minutes
Serves: 6
Ingredients:

- 12 eggs
- 2 cups cooked quinoa
- 1 teaspoon olive oil
- 1 teaspoon garlic powder
- 1 teaspoon onion powder
- 1/4 cup Greek yogurt
- 1 cup feta cheese, crumbled
- 2 cups cherry tomatoes, halved
- 5 ounces baby spinach
- 1/2 teaspoon pepper
- 1/2 teaspoon salt

Directions:

In a mixing bowl, whisk together eggs, yogurt, garlic powder, onion powder, pepper, and salt and set aside.

Heat oil in a large pan over medium heat.

Add spinach and sauté until spinach is wilted, about 3–4 minutes.

Add tomatoes and cook until tomatoes are softened.

Add egg mixture and stir until eggs are set, about 8–10 minutes.

Once the eggs are set, stir in quinoa and crumbled cheese and cook for 2–3 minutes.

Serve and enjoy.

Nutritional Data: 424 calories | 18.92g carbs | 26.69g fat | 26.21g protein | 655mg sodium

7- Egg-and-Veggie Muffins

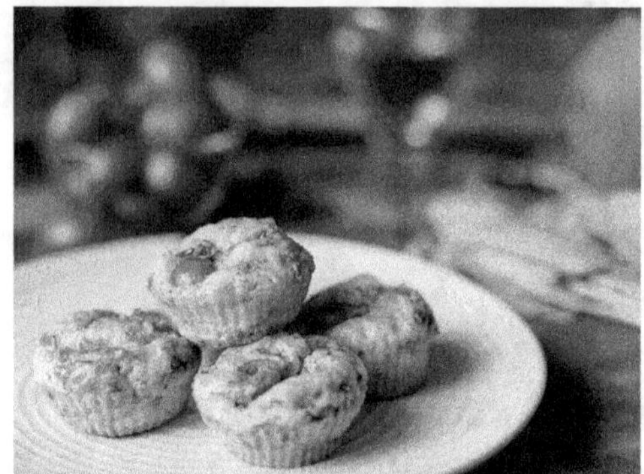

Preparation Time: 10 minutes
Cooking Time: 20 minutes
Serves: 12
Ingredients:

- 12 eggs
- 1 cup tomatoes, chopped
- 1/4 tsp garlic powder
- 1 cup baby spinach, chopped
- 1/2 tsp Italian seasoning
- 4 tbsp water
- Pepper
- Salt

Directions:

Preheat oven to 350°F.

Spray a muffin pan with cooking spray and set aside.

In a mixing bowl, whisk eggs with garlic powder, Italian seasoning, water, pepper, and salt.

Add tomatoes and spinach and stir well.

Pour egg mixture into the prepared muffin pan and bake for 20 minutes.

Serve and enjoy.

Nutritional Data: 138 calories | 2.52g carbs | 9.75g fat | 9.64g protein | 121mg sodium

8- Greek Yogurt Parfait

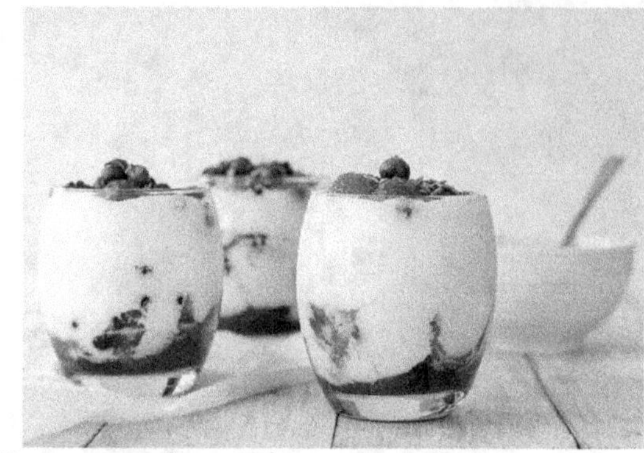

Preparation Time: 5 minutes
Cooking Time: 5 minutes
Serves: 4
Ingredients:

- 4 cups plain Greek yogurt
- 1/2 cup walnuts, toasted & chopped
- 8 dates, pitted & chopped
- 1/2 cup honey

Directions:

Add a spoonful of yogurt to the bottom of each of the four serving glasses.

Top with dates and walnuts. Drizzle with honey.

Repeat steps 1 and 2, and then end with an additional layer of honey. Place in the refrigerator until ready to serve.

Nutritional Data: 308 calories | 51.44g carbs | 7.06g fat | 14.74g protein | 47mg sodium

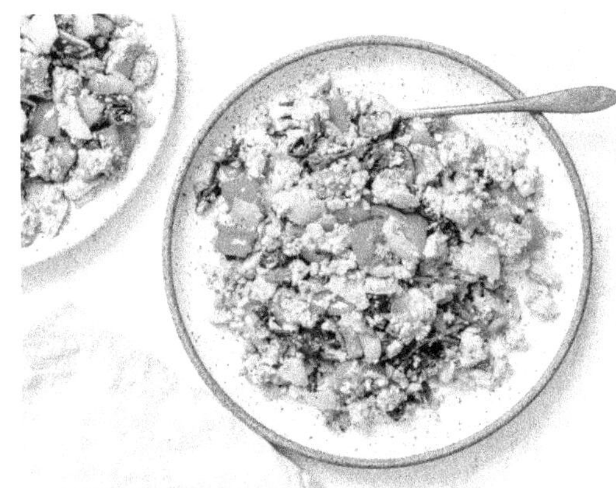

Preparation Time: 10 minutes
Cooking Time: 7 minutes
Serves: 2
Ingredients:

- 1/2 block firm tofu, crumbled
- 1 tbsp chives, chopped
- 1 tbsp coriander, chopped
- 1/4 tsp ground cumin
- 1/4 cup zucchini, chopped
- 1 tbsp turmeric
- 1 cup spinach
- 1 tbsp olive oil
- 1 medium tomato, chopped
- Pepper
- Salt

Directions:

Heat oil in a pan over medium heat.

Add zucchini, tomato, and spinach to the pan and sauté for 2 minutes.

Add tofu, cumin, turmeric, pepper, and salt, and sauté for 5 minutes.

Top with coriander and chives.

Serve and enjoy.

Nutritional Data: 170 calories | 10.55g carbs | 11.48g fat | 9.62g protein | 28mg sodium

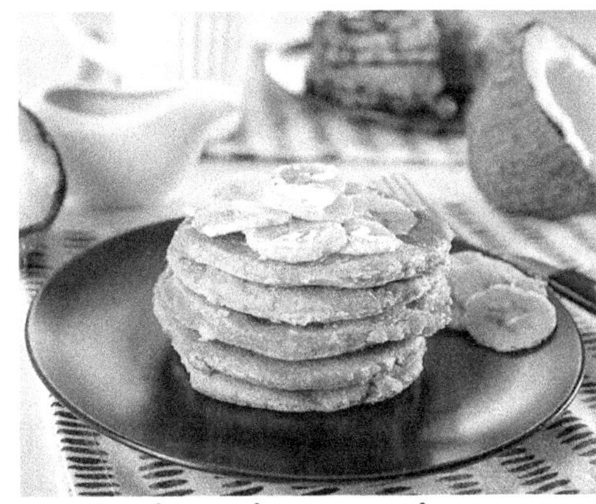

Preparation Time: 5 minutes
Cooking Time: 5 minutes
Serves: 1
Ingredients:

- 2 eggs
- 1 tbsp coconut flour
- 1/2 tsp vanilla
- 1 packet stevia
- 1/2 tsp cinnamon
- 2 oz cream cheese

Directions:

Add all ingredients into a bowl and blend until smooth.

Spray pan with cooking spray and heat over medium-high heat.

Pour batter on a hot pan and make two pancakes.

Cook pancake until lightly brown on both sides.

Serve and enjoy.

Nutritional Data: 438 calories | 6.88g carbs | 35.54g fat | 22.12g protein | 468mg sodium

11- Salmon-and-Avocado Wrap

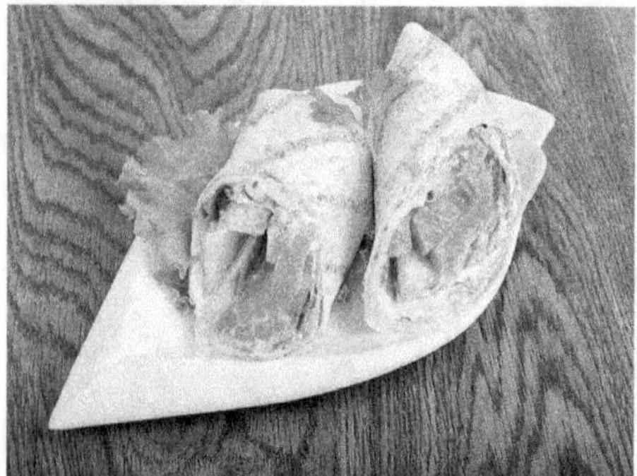

Preparation Time: 5 minutes
Cooking Time: 5 minutes
Serves: 2
Ingredients:
- 2 whole-wheat tortillas
- ½ lemon juice
- 1 cup watercress
- 1 avocado, sliced
- 2 tbsp cream cheese
- 2 smoked salmon slices
- Pepper
- Salt

Directions:

Warm up the tortillas in a pan for a minute then transfer them to a plate.

Spread cream cheese on tortilla then scatter some watercress on top.

Place avocado slices on top of watercress then place salmon slice. Drizzle with lemon juice and season with pepper and salt.

Roll up the wrap tightly and secure it with a toothpick.

Serve and enjoy.

Nutritional Data: 407 calories | 31.09g carbs | 25.98g fat | 16.21g protein | 464mg sodium

12- Green Smoothie

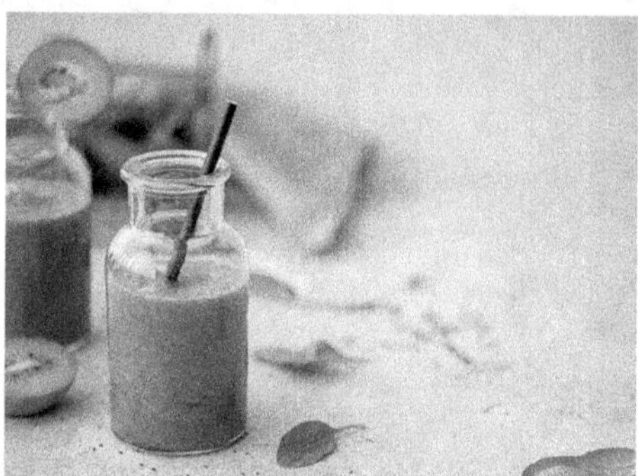

Preparation Time: 5 minutes
Cooking Time: 5 minutes
Serves: 2
Ingredients:
- 2 cups spinach leaves
- ¼ cup orange juice
- 1 tbsp almond butter
- 1 tbsp maple syrup
- ½ tsp vanilla
- 1 tbsp chia seeds
- Pinch of turmeric
- ¼ tsp spirulina powder
- ½ tsp cinnamon
- ½ banana
- ½ avocado
- 1 cup mango chunks
- 1 cup unsweetened almond milk

Directions:

Add spinach and remaining ingredients into blender and blend until smooth and creamy.

Serve and enjoy.

Nutritional Data: 319 calories | 48.26g carbs | 13.91g fat | 5.71g protein | 137mg sodium

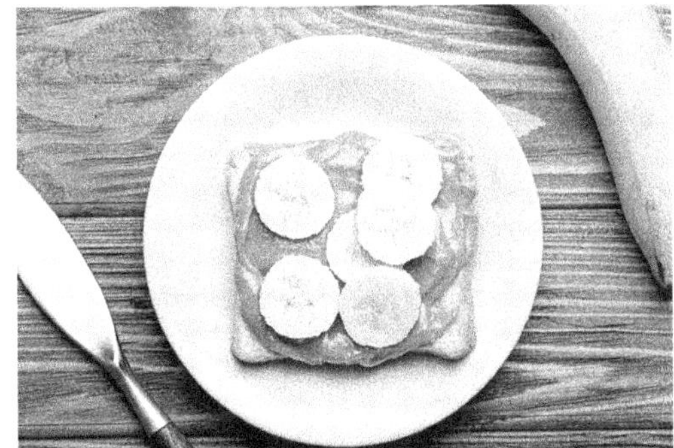

Preparation Time: 5 minutes
Cooking Time: 5 minutes
Serves: 2
Ingredients:

- 2 whole-wheat bread slices
- 1 banana, sliced
- 2 tbsp almonds, slivered
- 1 tbsp honey
- ½ tsp cinnamon
- 2 tbsp almond butter

Directions:

Place bread slices in a pan and toast them on medium heat.

Spread almond butter on toasted bread slices and top with sliced bananas. Sprinkle slivered almonds and cinnamon on top of banana slices.

Drizzle with honey and serve.

Nutritional Data: 361 calories | 61.12g carbs | 11.35g fat | 10.58g protein | 322mg sodium

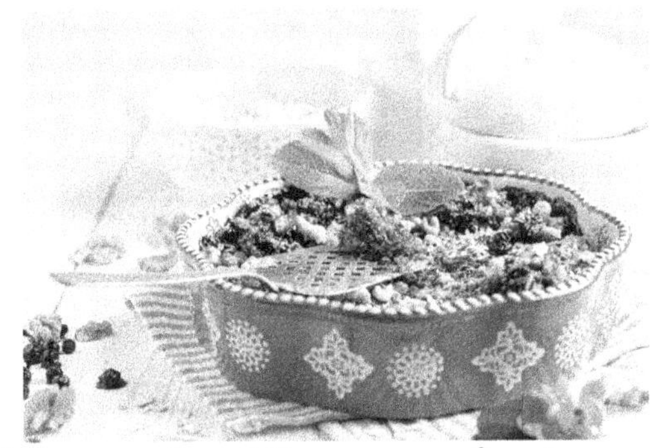

Preparation Time: 10 minutes
Cooking Time: 75 minutes
Serves: 8
Ingredients:

- 1 cup quinoa
- 1 tsp vanilla
- 2 tbsp maple syrup
- 2 flax eggs
- 2 cups coconut milk
- 1 tbsp ground cinnamon
- ½ cup strawberries
- ½ cup raspberries
- 1 cup blueberries

Directions:

Preheat oven to 375°F.

Add quinoa and remaining ingredients into baking dish and stir well to combine.

Bake in preheated oven for 65–75 minutes or until the quinoa is cooked. Remove from oven and allow to cool for 15 minutes.

Serve and enjoy.

Nutritional Data: 311 calories | 32.9g carbs | 18.17g fat | 7.06g protein | 38mg sodium

15- Cottage Cheese Bowl

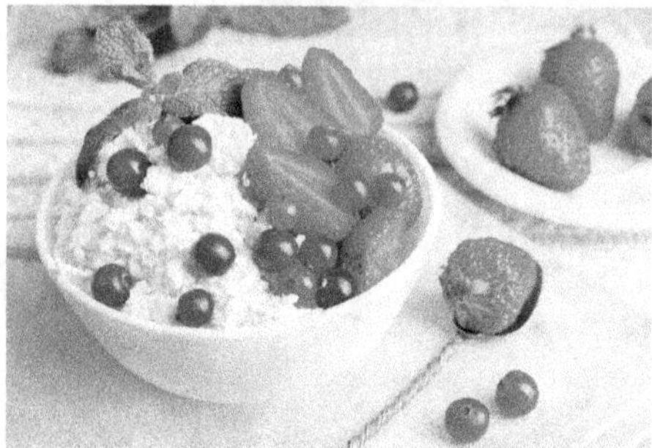

Preparation Time: 5 minutes
Cooking Time: 5 minutes
Serves: 2
Ingredients:

- 2 cups cottage cheese
- 1 tsp poppy seeds
- 1 tbsp honey
- ½ tsp lemon zest, grated
- 2 tbsp almonds, slivered
- 6 pineberries, sliced
- 6 strawberries, sliced
- 15 basil leaves, sliced

Directions:

Mix together cottage cheese and basil.

Transfer the cottage cheese mixture into two serving bowls.

Top each bowl with sliced strawberries, pineberries, slivered almonds, and lemon zest. Sprinkle with poppy seeds.

Drizzle with honey and serve.

Nutritional Data: 496 calories | 19.35g carbs | 30.6g fat | 36.63g protein | 817mg sodium

16 Egg-and-Veggie Stir-Fry

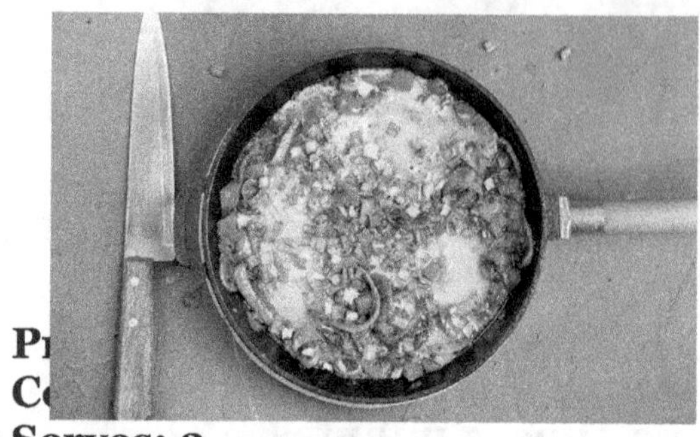

Preparation Time:
Cooking Time:
Serves: 2
Ingredients:

- 4 eggs, lightly beaten
- 1 tbsp olive oil
- 1/2 cup cheddar cheese, shredded
- 1 tsp garlic, minced
- 1 cup fresh spinach
- 2 cups chard, stemmed & chopped
- 1/2 cup arugula
- Pepper
- Salt
- 1 cup blueberries

Directions:

Heat oil in a pan over medium-high heat.

Add spinach, arugula, and chard and sauté for 3 minutes.

Add garlic and sauté for a minute.

In a bowl, whisk eggs with cheese and pour over the veggie mixture.

Cover and cook for 5–7 minutes. Season with pepper and salt.

Serve and enjoy.

Nutritional Data: 389 calories | 9.59g carbs | 28.64g fat | 23.3g protein | 594mg sodium

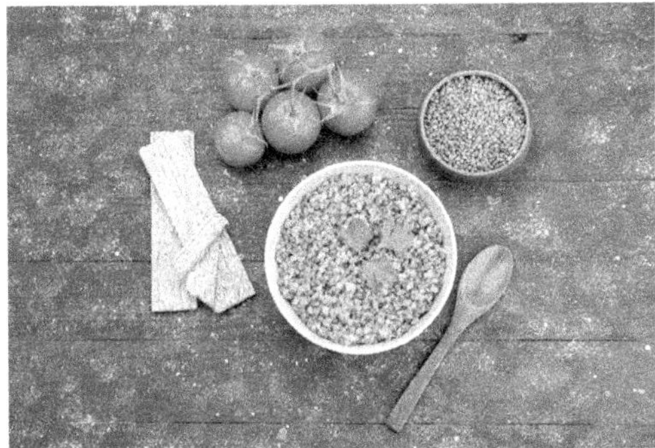

Preparation Time: 5 minutes
Cooking Time: 6 minutes
Serves: 2
Ingredients:

- 1 cup buckwheat groats, rinsed
- 3 cups unsweetened almond milk
- 1 tsp ground cinnamon
- 1 banana, sliced
- Pinch of salt

Directions:

Spray instant pot from the inside with cooking spray.

Add all ingredients into instant pot and stir well.

Seal instant pot with a lid and cook on high pressure for 6 minutes.

Once done, release pressure manually. Remove lid.

Stir well and serve.

Nutritional Data: 313 calories | 65.04g carbs | 5.23g fat | 5.8g protein | 260mg sodium

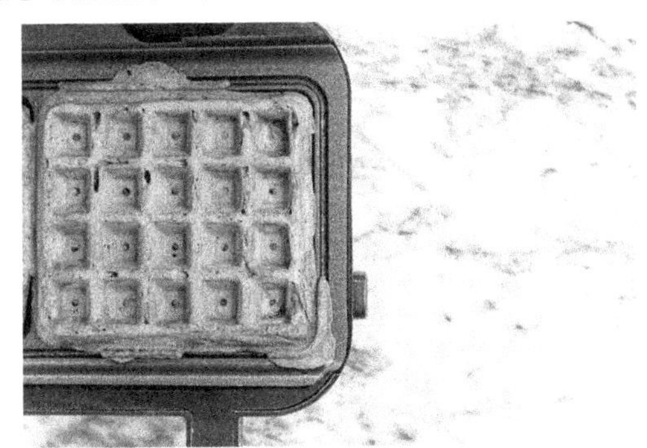

Preparation Time: 5 minutes
Cooking Time: 5 minutes
Serves: 1
Ingredients:

- 1 egg
- 2 tbsp almond flour
- 1 oz cream cheese
- 1 1/2 tsp monk fruit
- 1 tsp vanilla
- 1 tbsp cocoa powder

Directions:

Preheat waffle maker.

In a bowl, whisk egg with vanilla. Add remaining ingredients and mix well.

Spray the waffle maker with cooking spray.

Pour 1/3 cup of batter onto the center of the waffle square.

Lower the lid and cook until the waffle is lightly golden on both sides.

Serve and enjoy.

Nutritional Data: 257 calories | 7.68g carbs | 19.68g fat | 12.5g protein | 228mg sodium

19-Mango Coconut Chia Pudding

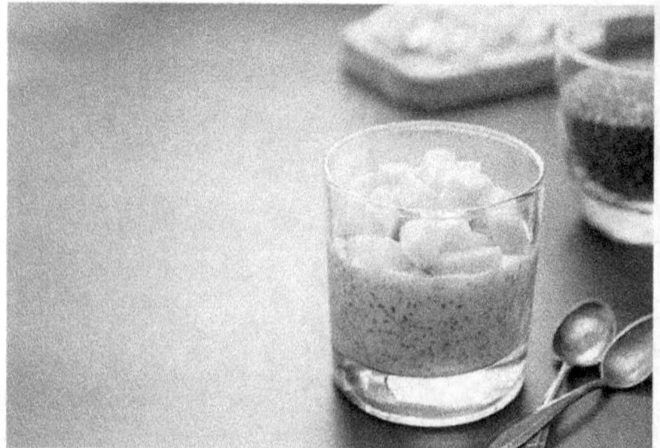

Preparation Time: 5 minutes
Cooking Time: 5 minutes
Serves: 2
Ingredients:

- 4 tbsp chia seeds
- 2 tbsp honey
- 1 tbsp shredded coconut
- ¾ cup fresh mango, diced
- ½ cup unsweetened almond milk
- ½ cup coconut milk

Directions:

Add chia seeds and remaining ingredients into mixing bowl and mix well. Cover and place in refrigerator overnight.

Stir well and serve

Nutritional Data: 147 calories | 17.69g carbs | 8.58g fat | 2.27g protein | 26mg sodium

20-Sardine Toast

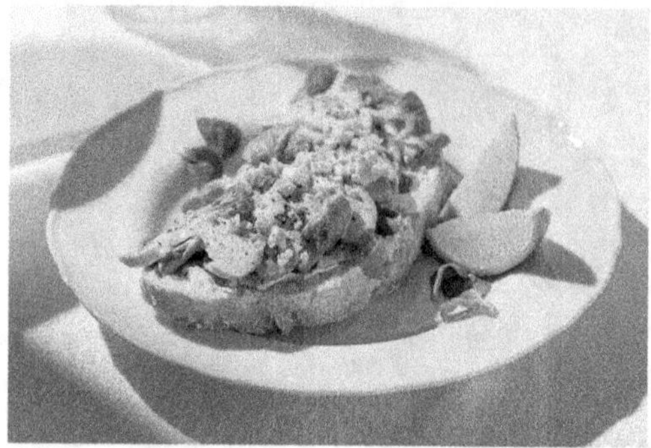

Preparation Time: 10 minutes
Cooking Time: 5 minutes
Serves: 4
Ingredients:

- 8.75-oz can of sardines, drained
- 4 whole-grain bread slices, toasted
- 1 ½ tbsp vegan mayonnaise
- 1 ½ tbsp ketchup
- ¼ cup parsley, chopped
- 2 shallots, chopped
- 4 radishes, finely chopped
- 2 dill pickles, chopped
- Pepper
- Salt

Directions:

In a bowl, mix together sardines, mayonnaise, ketchup, parsley, shallots, radishes, dill pickle, pepper, and salt until well combined.

Spread the sardine mixture on top of each toasted bread slice.

Serve and enjoy.

Nutritional Data: 341 calories | 37.31g carbs | 11.23g fat | 23.98g protein | 1068mg sodium

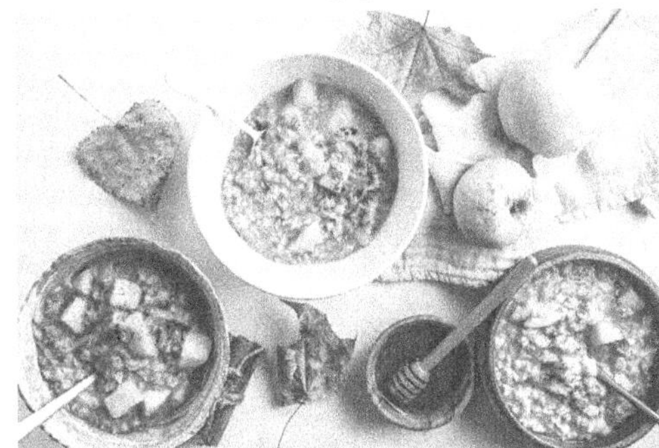

Preparation Time: 5 minutes
Cooking Time: 10 minutes
Serves: 4
Ingredients:

- 2 cups rolled oats
- 1 tsp ground cinnamon
- 2 apples, cored & diced
- 3 tbsp maple syrup
- 1 cup fresh apple cider
- 2 ½ cups water
- ¼ tsp salt

Directions:

Add apple cider, apples, maple syrup, water, and salt to a medium pot and bring to a boil over medium-high heat.

Once boiling begins, turn heat to medium-low. Add cinnamon and oats and cook for 3–5 minutes.

Serve and enjoy.

Nutritional Data: 232 calories | 61.28g carbs | 3.56g fat | 8.46g protein | 155mg sodium

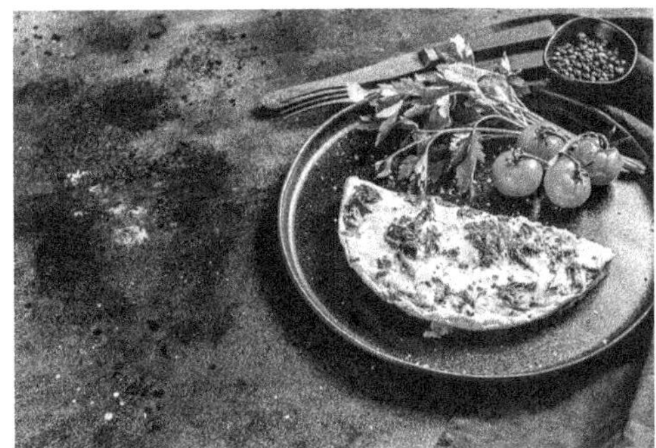

Preparation Time: 5 minutes
Cooking Time: 10 minutes
Serves: 1
Ingredients:

- 3 eggs
- 1 tbsp water
- 1 cup baby spinach
- 1 cup mushrooms, sliced
- 2 tbsp olive oil
- ¼ tsp pepper
- ¼ tsp salt

Directions:

Heat 1 tablespoon of oil in a pan over medium heat.

Add mushrooms and cook for 5 minutes. Season with pepper and salt.

Add spinach and cook for 1–2 minutes or until it is wilted.

Transfer mushroom-spinach mixture to a plate.

In a bowl, whisk eggs with 1 tablespoon of water, pepper, and salt.

Heat the remaining oil in the same pan over medium heat.

Add egg mixture and cook for 1 minute or until eggs are set.

Add mushroom-spinach mixture on top of the omelet, fold the omelet in half, and transfer to a plate.

Serve and enjoy.

Nutritional Data: 640 calories | 5.4g carbs | 56.08g fat | 28.17g protein | 914mg sodium

23-Pumpkin Smoothie

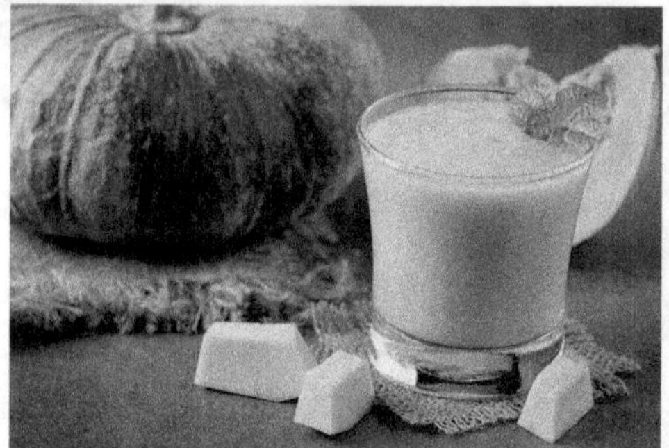

Preparation Time: 5 minutes
Cooking Time: 5 minutes
Serves: 1
Ingredients:

- ½ cup pumpkin puree
- 1 scoop vanilla protein powder
- ½ tsp turmeric
- ½ tsp pumpkin pie spice
- 1 tbsp cashew butter
- 1 cup unsweetened almond milk

Directions:

Add pumpkin puree and remaining ingredients into blender.

Blend until smooth and creamy.

Serve immediately and enjoy.

Nutritional Data: 738 calories | 50.67g carbs | 43.09g fat | 46.26g protein | 699mg sodium

24-Tomato Basil Avocado Toast

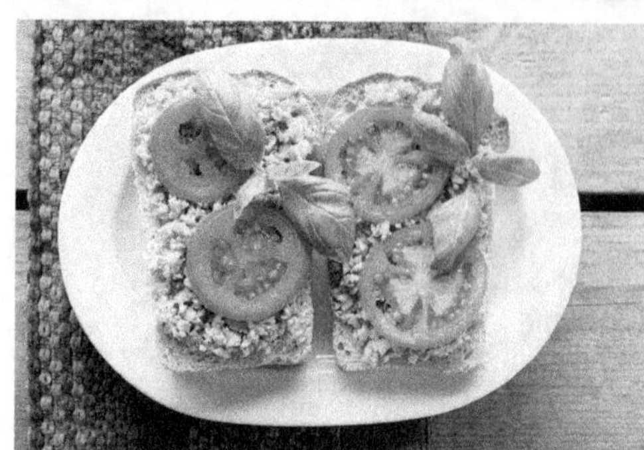

Preparation Time: 10 minutes
Cooking Time: 10 minutes
Serves: 2
Ingredients:

- 2 whole-grain bread slices, toasted
- 10 grape tomatoes, cut in half
- 1 avocado, flesh scooped out
- 1 tbsp olive oil
- 8 basil leaves, sliced
- Pepper
- Salt

Directions:

Add avocado flesh in a bowl. Mash using a fork. Season with pepper and salt.

Spread mashed avocado onto the toasted bread slices.

Top with tomatoes and basil. Drizzle with olive oil.

Serve and enjoy.

Nutritional Data: 355 calories | 32.96g carbs | 23.31g fat | 8.18g protein | 166mg sodium

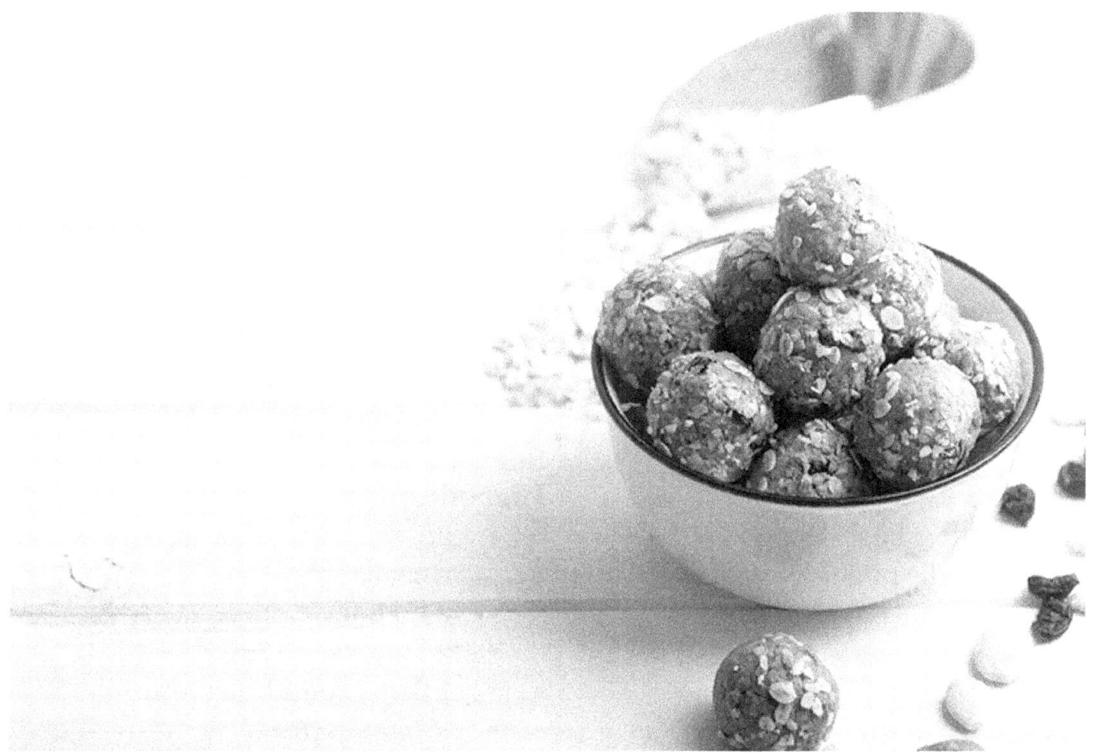

Preparation Time: 10 minutes
Cooking Time: 15 minutes
Serves: 18 balls
Ingredients:
- ½ cup vanilla protein powder
- 1 cup creamy almond butter
- 1 tsp vanilla
- ½ tsp cinnamon
- ½ cup unsweetened chocolate chips
- 1 cup quick oats
- 1/3 cup honey
- 1/8 tsp salt

Directions:

In a mixing bowl, mix together protein powder, almond butter, vanilla, cinnamon, chocolate chips, oats, honey, and salt until well combined.

Make equal shapes of balls from the oat mixture and place onto parchment-lined plate. Place in the refrigerator for 60 minutes to set.

Serve and enjoy.

Nutritional Data: 159 calories | 14.82g carbs | 9.33g fat | 5.92g protein | 77mg sodium

Chapter 3 —Appetizer Recipes

1-Guacamole with Veggie Sticks

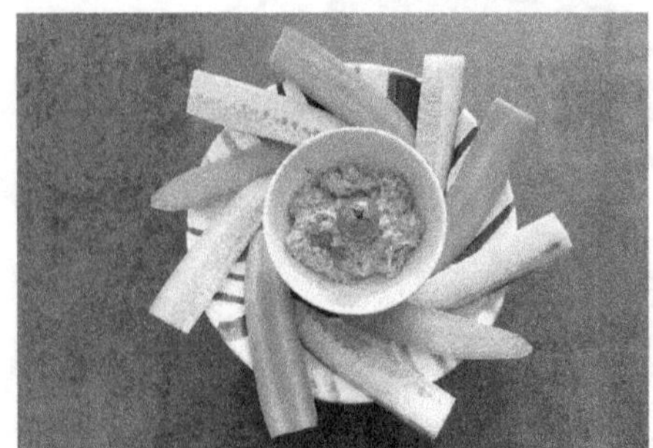

Preparation Time: 10 minutes
Cooking Time: 5 minutes
Serves: 6
Ingredients:

- 2 avocados, flesh scooped out
- ½ tsp garlic powder
- 1 tsp hot sauce
- 1 tbsp lime juice
- 2 tbsp cilantro, chopped
- 1 tomato, chopped
- 1/3 cup onion, chopped
- Pepper
- Salt

Directions:

Add avocado flesh into bowl and mash using a fork.

Add onion, tomato, cilantro, lime juice, hot sauce, garlic powder, pepper, and salt and mix well.

Serve guacamole with veggie sticks

Nutritional Data: 118 calories | 8.25g carbs | 9.89g fat | 1.81g protein | 28mg sodium

2-Turmeric Hummus

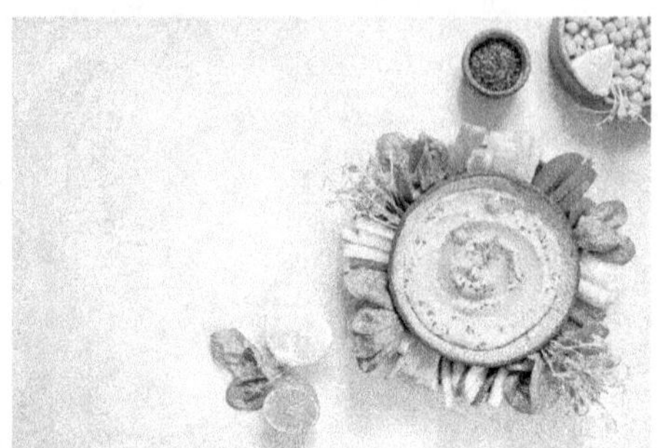

Preparation Time: 5 minutes
Cooking Time: 5 minutes
Serves: 8
Ingredients:

- 28-oz can chickpeas, drained & rinsed
- 2 tbsp olive oil
- 2 lemons, juiced
- 1 tbsp ground turmeric
- ½ cup tahini
- 2 garlic cloves
- ½ tsp pepper
- ½ tsp sea salt

Directions:

Add chickpeas and remaining ingredients into food processor and process until smooth and creamy.

Serve and enjoy.

Nutritional Data: 265 calories | 28g carbs | 13.97g fat | 9.8g protein | 374mg sodium

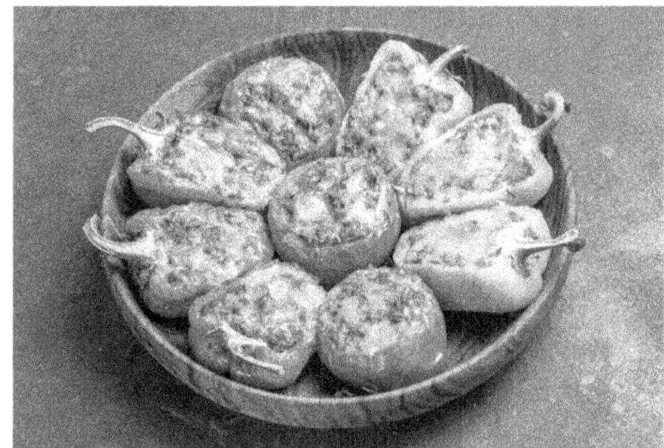

Preparation Time: 10 minutes
Cooking Time: 25 minutes
Serves: 4
Ingredients:

- 4 eggs
- 2 bell peppers, cut in half and deseeded
- 1/4 cup baby broccoli florets
- 1/4 cup cherry tomatoes
- 1 tsp dried sage
- 2.5 oz cheddar cheese, grated
- 7 oz unsweetened almond milk
- Pepper
- Salt

Directions:

In a bowl, mix together eggs, cherry tomatoes, sage, milk, broccoli, pepper, and salt.

Pour egg mixture into the bell pepper halves.

Sprinkle cheese on top of bell pepper.

Place stuffed bell pepper into the baking dish and bake at 390°F for 25 minutes.

Serve and enjoy

Nutritional Data: 437 calories | 32.87g carbs | 28.39g fat | 16.59g protein | 337mg sodium

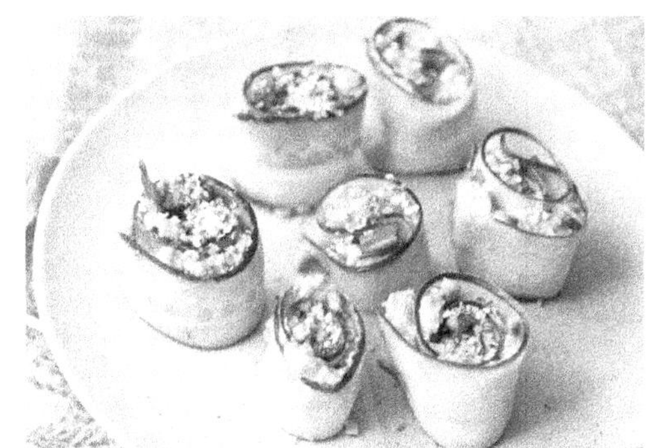

Preparation Time: 10 minutes
Cooking Time: 5 minutes
Serves: 20 rolls
Ingredients:

- 1 English cucumber, sliced into thin strips using a peeler
- 1 avocado, flesh scooped out
- 1 garlic clove
- 2 tsp lime juice
- 1 tbsp nutritional yeast
- ¼ cup fresh basil
- ¼ tsp pepper
- ¼ tsp salt

Directions:

Add avocado flesh, garlic, lime juice, nutritional yeast, basil, pepper, and salt into food processor and process until smooth.

Transfer avocado mixture into bowl.

Place one strip of cucumber on the cutting board then spread some avocado mixture on the cucumber strip and roll. Make the remaining cucumber strip rolls.

Serve and enjoy.

Nutritional Data: 18 calories | 1.2g carbs | 1.49g fat | 0.45g protein | 57mg sodium

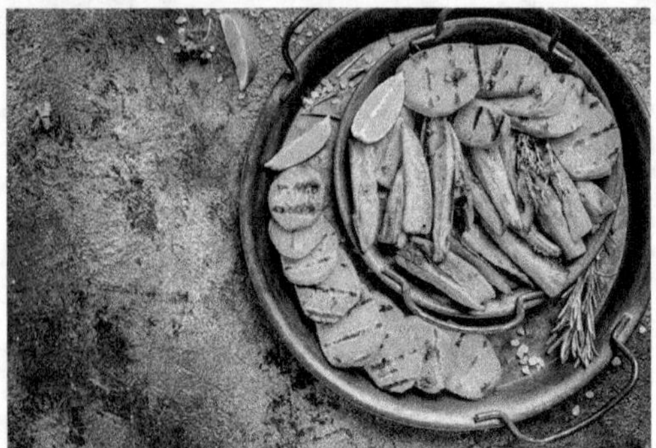

Preparation Time: 10 minutes
Cooking Time: 15 minutes
Serves: 2
Ingredients:

- 2 sweet potatoes, peeled and cut into fries
- 1/4 tsp paprika
- 1/2 tsp chili powder
- 1 tbsp olive oil
- 1/4 tsp garlic powder
- Salt

Directions:

In a bowl, toss sweet potato fries with chili powder, garlic powder, paprika, olive oil, and salt until well coated.

Spread sweet potato fries onto the baking sheet.

Bake sweet potato fries at 380°F for 15 minutes.

Serve and enjoy.

Nutritional Data: 139 calories | 16.68g carbs | 7.81g fat | 4.68g protein | 31mg sodium

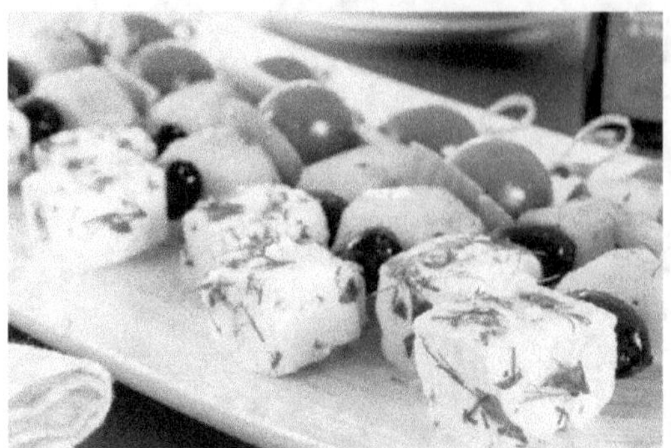

Preparation Time: 10 minutes
Cooking Time: 5 minutes
Serves: 6
Ingredients:

- 12 olives, pitted
- 12 grape tomatoes
- 8 oz feta cheese, cut into 12 pieces
- 1 cucumber, cut into 12 slices
- ½ tsp Italian seasoning
- 1 tbsp olive oil
- Pepper
- Salt

Directions:

Thread one olive, grape tomato, feta cheese, and cucumber slice on a wooden skewer.

Place salad skewers on a plate and drizzle with olive oil and sprinkle with Italian seasoning.

Season salad skewers with pepper and salt.

Serve and enjoy.

Nutritional Data: 138 calories | 4.4g carbs | 11.15g fat | 5.66g protein | 448mg sodium

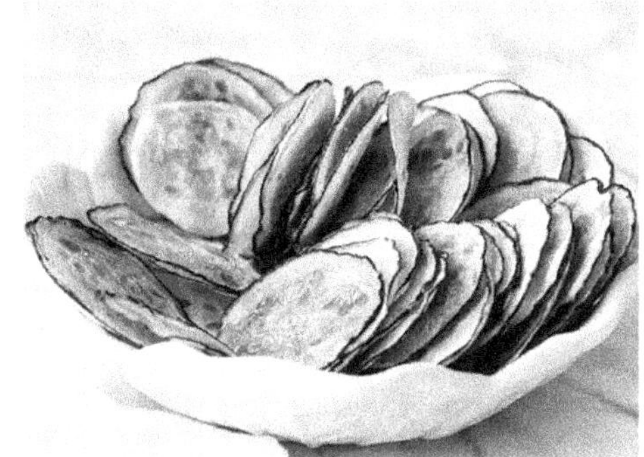

Preparation Time: 5 minutes
Cooking Time: 5 minutes
Serves: 2
Ingredients:
- 2 zucchinis, cut into 1/4-inch-thick slices
- 2 tsp olive oil
- 1/2 tsp sea salt

Directions:

In a mixing bowl, toss zucchini slices with oil, and salt.

Arrange zucchini slices into the air fryer basket and cook at 350°F for 10 minutes.

Serve and enjoy.

Nutritional Data: 42 calories | 0.34g carbs | 4.54g fat | 0.3g protein | 582mg sodium

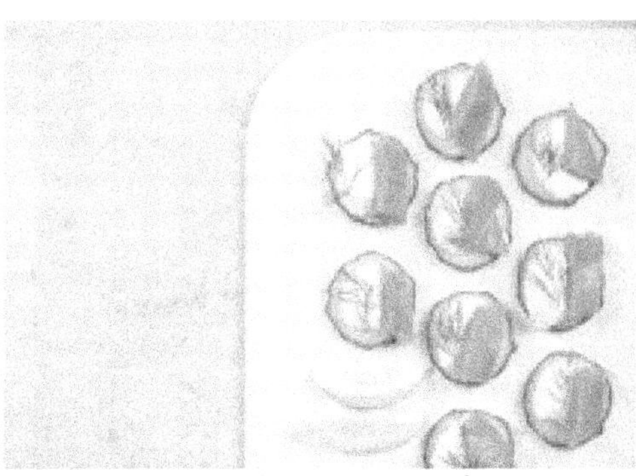

Preparation Time: 10 minutes
Cooking Time: 5 minutes
Serves: 32 bites
Ingredients:
- 1 large cucumber, sliced into ½-inch rounds
- 1 garlic clove, chopped
- 8 oz smoked salmon, cut into bite-size pieces
- 3 tbsp chives, chopped
- 1 tsp fresh lemon juice
- 4 oz cream cheese
- Pepper
- Salt

Directions:

In a bowl, mix together cream cheese, 1 tablespoon of chives, garlic, lemon juice, pepper, and salt.

Spread some cream cheese on top of each cucumber slice and top with a salmon piece.

Garnish with the rest of the chopped chives.

Serve and enjoy.

Nutritional Data: 22 calories | 0.32g carbs | 1.53g fat | 1.76g protein | 46mg sodium

9-Stuffed Mushrooms

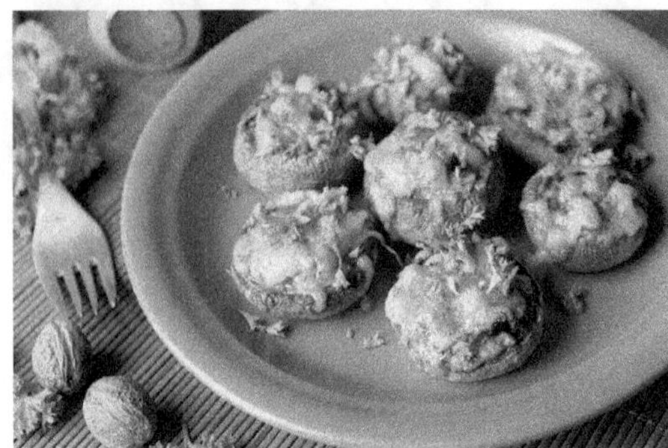

Preparation Time: 10 minutes
Cooking Time: 8 minutes
Serves: 4
Ingredients:

- 16 oz button mushrooms, cleaned & stems cut
- 3 tbsp sour cream
- 6 oz cream cheese, softened
- 1/2 tsp garlic powder
- 1/4 cup cheddar cheese, shredded
- Pepper
- Salt

Directions:

In a small bowl, mix together cream cheese, sour cream, garlic powder, pepper, and salt.

Stuff cream cheese mixture into each mushroom cap and top each with cheddar cheese.

Place stuff mushrooms into the air fryer basket and cook at 370°F for 8–10 minutes.

Serve and enjoy.

Nutritional Data: 504 calories | 90.48g carbs | 15.53g fat | 16.4g protein | 366mg sodium

10-Edamame Salad

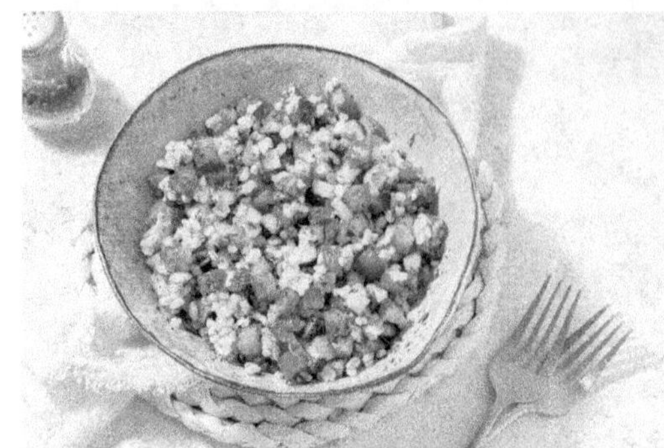

Preparation Time: 10 minutes
Cooking Time: 5 minutes
Serves: 4
Ingredients:

- 12 oz shelled edamame
- 2 tsp sesame seeds
- ¼ cup cilantro, chopped
- 2 green onions, sliced
- 1 red bell pepper, diced
- 1 cup cucumber, chopped
- For dressing:
- 2 tbsp rice wine vinegar
- ¼ tsp ground ginger
- ½ tsp sriracha
- 2 tsp maple syrup
- 1 tsp low-sodium soy sauce
- 1 tsp sesame oil
- 2 tsp olive oil

Directions:

In a mixing bowl, mix together edamame, sesame seeds, cilantro, green onion, bell pepper, and cucumber.

In a small bowl, mix together all dressing ingredients and pour over salad.

Toss well and serve immediately.

Nutritional Data: 166 calories | 13.38g carbs | 8.98g fat | 10.12g protein | 29mg sodium

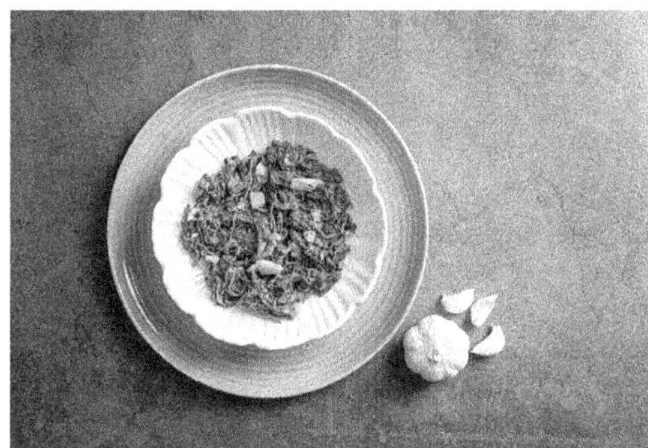

Preparation Time: 10 minutes
Cooking Time: 15 minutes
Serves: 6
Ingredients:

- 1 3/4 lbs kale, rinsed and chopped
- 1 tbsp garlic, minced
- 1 tbsp fresh lime juice
- 2 tbsp onion, minced
- 1 tbsp olive oil
- Salt

Directions:

Heat oil in a large pan over medium-high heat.

Add onion and garlic and sauté for 1–2 minutes.

Add kale and sauté for 5 minutes or until wilted. Cover and cook for 6–8 minutes.

Remove the cover and cook for 2 minutes more.

Add lime juice and stir well.

Serve and enjoy.

Nutritional Data: 89 calories | 12.57g carbs | 3.49g fat | 5.8g protein | 51mg sodium

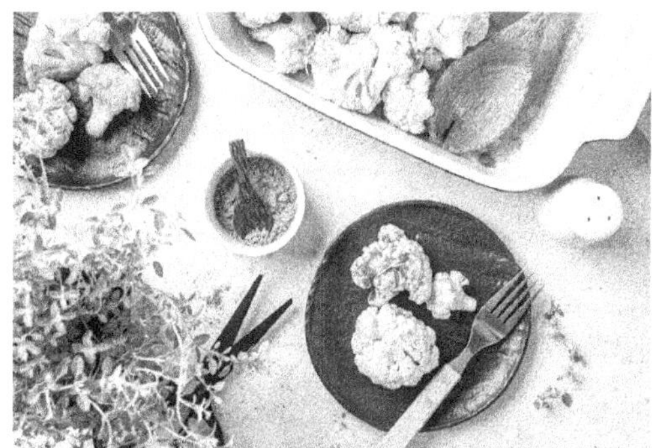

Preparation Time: 10 minutes
Cooking Time: 30 minutes
Serves: 4
Ingredients:

- 1 large cauliflower head, cut into florets
- ½ tsp cayenne powder
- ½ tsp turmeric
- ½ tsp cumin powder
- 2 tsp curry powder
- 1 tbsp lime juice
- 1 tbsp olive oil
- ½ tsp sea salt

Directions:

Preheat oven to 425°F.

Line baking sheet with parchment paper and set aside.

Add cauliflower florets and remaining ingredients into large mixing bowl and toss until well coated.

Spread cauliflower florets onto baking sheet and bake in preheated oven for 30 minutes.

Serve and enjoy.

Nutritional Data: 54 calories | 4.67g carbs | 3.82g fat | 1.54g protein | 312mg sodium

13-Cilantro Lime Shrimp Skewers

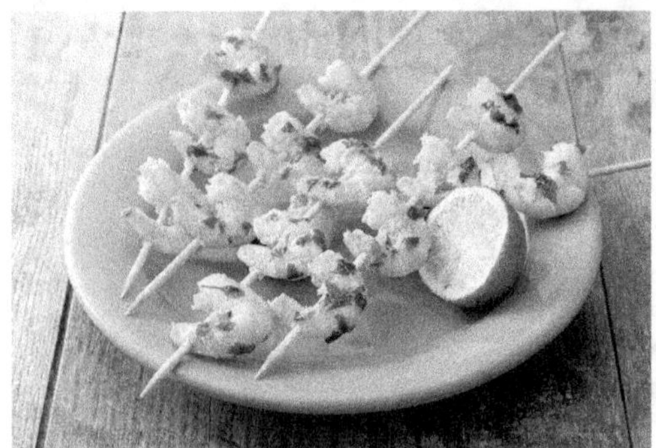

Preparation Time: 10 minutes
Cooking Time: 10 minutes
Serves: 6
Ingredients:

- 1 1/2 lbs shrimp, deveined
- 2 tbsp fresh cilantro, chopped
- 2 tsp garlic paste
- 1/4 cup olive oil
- 1 tsp sweet paprika
- 2 fresh lime juice
- 1/2 tbsp dried oregano
- Pepper
- Salt

Directions:

Add shrimp and remaining ingredients into mixing bowl and mix well.

Cover and place in the refrigerator for 2 hours.

Thread marinated shrimp onto the soaked wooden skewers.

Preheat the grill to medium heat.

Place shrimp skewers on a hot grill and cook for 5–7 minutes. Turn halfway through.

Serve and enjoy.

Nutritional Data: 202 calories | 2.47g carbs | 10.62g fat | 23.49g protein | 988mg sodium

14-Roasted Red Pepper Dip

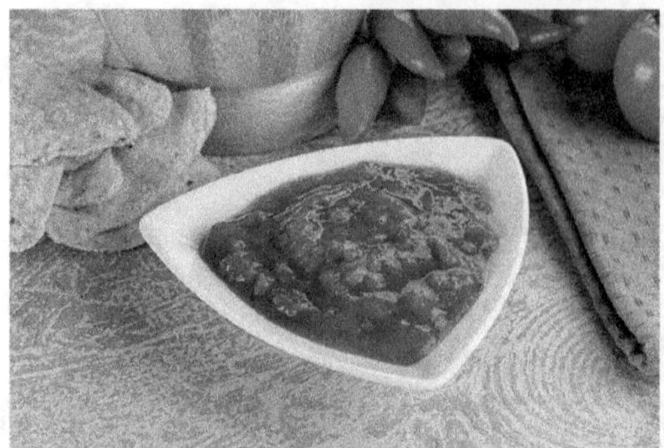

Preparation Time: 5 minutes
Cooking Time: 5 minutes
Serves: 20
Ingredients:

- 1 cup roasted red peppers
- ¼ tsp red pepper flakes, crushed
- 1 tsp lime juice
- ½ tsp dried basil
- 8 oz cream cheese
- 1 tsp garlic, minced

Directions:

Add roasted red peppers and remaining ingredients into blender and blend until smooth and creamy.

Serve and enjoy.

Nutritional Data: 36 calories | 0.98g carbs | 3.26g fat | 0.89g protein | 50mg sodium

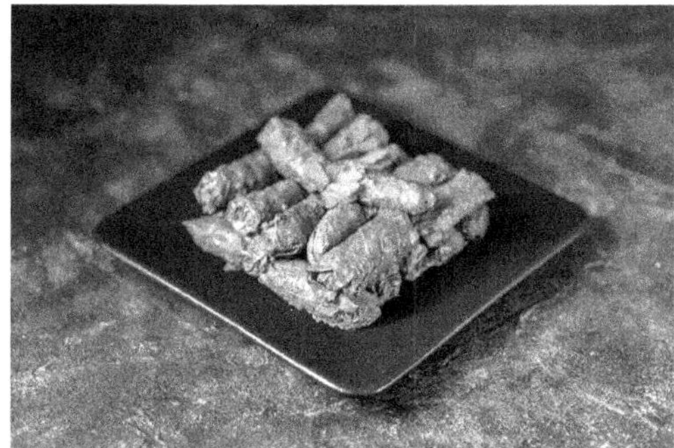

Preparation Time: 15 minutes
Cooking Time: 60 minutes
Serves: 8
Ingredients:

- 1 jar grape leaves, boiled in water for 10 minutes & drained well
- 1 cup cooked quinoa
- 3 tbsp apple butter
- 1 cup cooked brown rice
- Salt
- For sauce:
- 1 cup apricot jelly, no sugar added
- ½ cup apricot, chopped
- 2 tsp dried mint
- ½ cup water
- ¾ cup lemon juice
- Salt

Directions:

In a bowl, mix together cooked quinoa, brown rice, apple butter, and salt until well combined.

Roll each grape leaves with 3 tablespoons of quinoa rice filling.

Place five grape leaves in the bottom of a large pot then place stuffed grape leaves in the pot.

Mix together all sauce ingredients and pour over the stuffed grapes leaves.

Place one plate upside down on the stuffed grape leaves and cover with a lid.

Place pot on heat and cook over high heat until the water starts simmering. Turn heat to low and simmer for 45–60 minutes.

Serve and enjoy.

Nutritional Data: 351 calories | 70.78g carbs | 3.3g fat | 12.05g protein | 457mg sodium

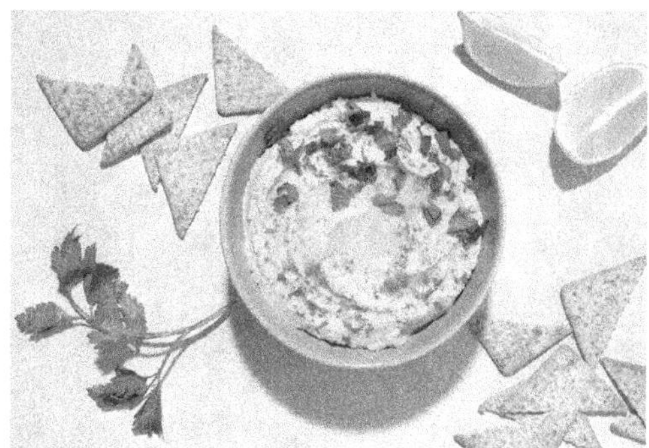

Preparation Time: 10 minutes
Cooking Time: 60 minutes
Serves: 6
Ingredients:

- 1 eggplant, peeled & diced
- 1/4 cup fresh parsley, chopped
- 3 tbsp lemon juice
- 1/2 tsp olive oil
- 3 garlic cloves, minced
- 1 tbsp tahini
- Pepper
- Salt

Directions:

Add eggplant and remaining ingredients into instant pot and stir well.

Cover, then select slow cook mode and cook on high for 1 hour.

Mash the eggplant mixture using a masher until desired consistency.

Serve and enjoy.

Nutritional Data: 49 calories | 7.79g carbs | 1.95g fat | 1.67g protein | 7mg sodium

17-Seaweed Salad

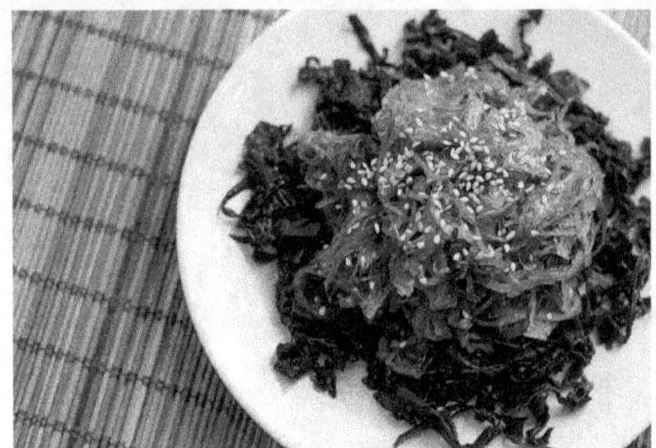

Preparation Time: 5 minutes
Cooking Time: 5 minutes
Serves: 4
Ingredients:

- 4 oz dried seaweed
- 1 tbsp sesame seeds
- 1 tsp ginger, grated
- 3 tbsp rice vinegar
- 1 tbsp sesame oil
- 3 tbsp low-sodium soy sauce
- 1 tbsp miso paste

Directions:

Soak seaweed in water for 5 minutes. Drain and rinse the seaweed and transfer it to a large bowl.

Mix together miso paste, ginger, sesame oil, vinegar, and soy sauce and pour over seaweed salad. Toss well to coat.

Sprinkle with sesame seeds and serve.

Nutritional Data: 96 calories | 6.44g carbs | 7.05g fat | 1.92g protein | 343mg sodium

18-Cauliflower Tabbouleh

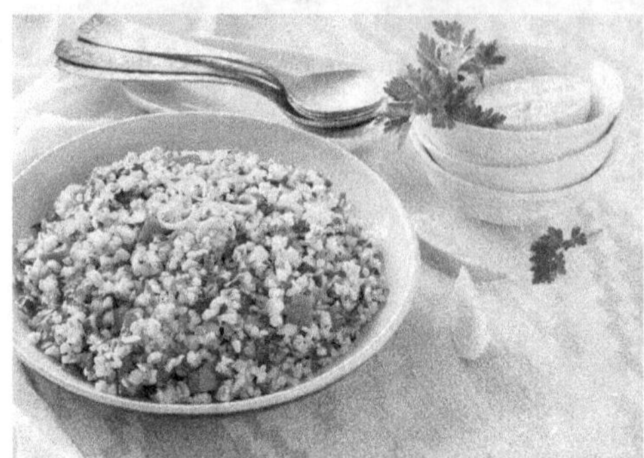

Preparation Time: 10 minutes
Cooking Time: 5 minutes
Serves: 4
Ingredients:

- 1/2 cauliflower head, grated
- 1 cup parsley, chopped
- 2 tbsp fresh lemon juice
- 2 tbsp fresh mint, chopped
- 2 green onions, chopped
- 1 tomato, chopped
- 1/4 cup olive oil
- 1/8 tsp pepper
- 1/4 tsp salt

Directions:

Add grated cauliflower and remaining ingredients into mixing bowl and mix well.

Serve and enjoy.

Nutritional Data: 314 calories | 6.5g carbs | 22.64g fat | 21.86g protein | 214mg sodium

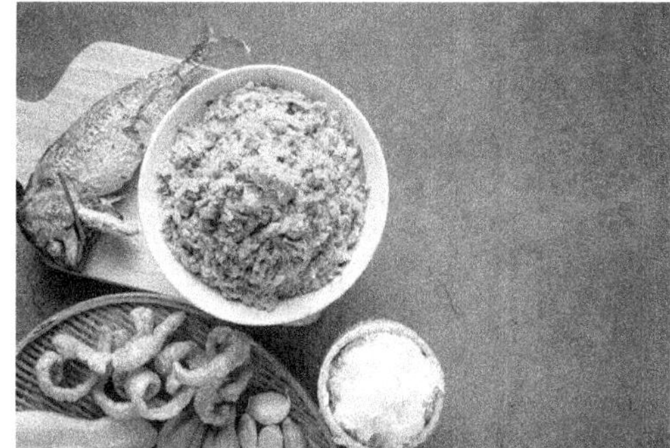

Preparation Time: 10 minutes
Cooking Time: 60 minutes
Serves: 6
Ingredients:

- 10-oz can artichoke hearts, drained & chopped
- 4 cups spinach, chopped
- 8 oz cream cheese
- 3 tbsp sour cream
- 1/4 cup mayonnaise
- 3/4 cup mozzarella cheese, shredded
- 1/4 cup parmesan cheese, grated
- 3 garlic cloves, minced
- 1/2 tsp dried parsley
- Pepper
- Salt

Directions:

Add all ingredients into slow cooker and stir well.

Cover and cook on low for 1 hour.

Stir well and serve.

Nutritional Data: 224 calories | 10.71g carbs | 16.05g fat | 11.34g protein | 472mg sodium

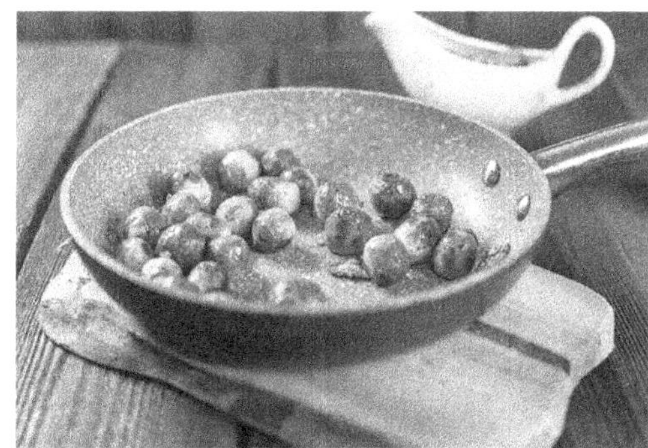

Preparation Time: 10 minutes
Cooking Time: 10 minutes
Serves: 8
Ingredients:

- 2 lbs Brussels sprouts, ends trimmed & shredded
- 1 tbsp olive oil
- 8 tsp pine nuts, toasted
- 1/4 cup basil, minced
- 2 tbsp lemon juice
- 3 medium shallots, minced
- 1/4 tsp pepper
- 2 tsp kosher salt

Directions:

Heat oil in a pan over medium-high heat.

Add shallots and sauté for 2 minutes.

Add Brussels sprouts and sauté for 5 minutes.

Stir in lemon juice, pine nuts, basil, pepper and salt.

Serve and enjoy.

Nutritional Data: 125 calories | 20.38g carbs | 4.02g fat | 5.69g protein | 617mg sodium

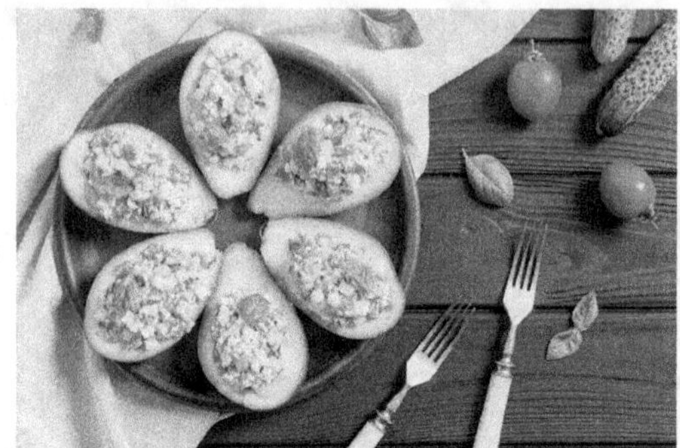

Preparation Time: 10 minutes
Cooking Time: 10 minutes
Serves: 2
Ingredients:

- 1 avocado, peeled, pitted & cut in half
- 1 tbsp balsamic vinegar
- 4 basil leaves, sliced
- ¼ cup grape tomatoes, cut in half
- ¼ cup mozzarella pearls
- Pepper
- Salt

Directions:

Place avocado halves onto a plate.

In a small bowl, mix together grape tomatoes, mozzarella pearls, and basil.

Spoon the tomato cheese mixture into each avocado half and drizzle with vinegar. Season with pepper and salt.

Serve and enjoy.

Nutritional Data: 278 calories | 34.94g carbs | 15.1g fat | 5.14g protein | 13mg sodium

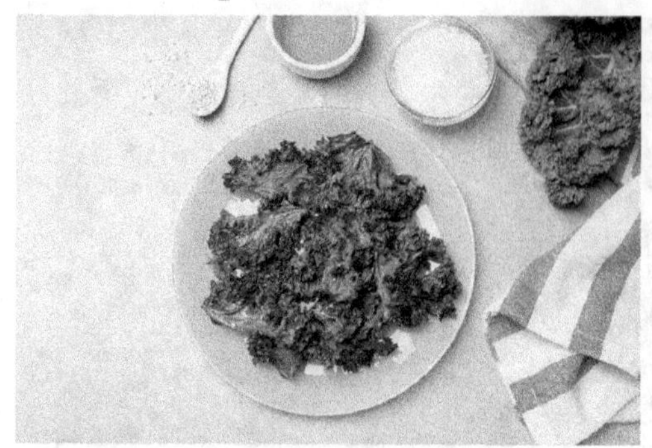

Preparation Time: 5 minutes
Cooking Time: 5 minutes
Serves: 2
Ingredients:

- 1 bunch of kale, stem removed & cut into pieces
- 1 tsp olive oil
- 1/2 tsp salt

Directions:

Add kale, oil, and salt into large bowl and toss well.

Transfer kale to air fryer basket and air-fry at 370°F for 5 minutes.

Serve and enjoy.

Nutritional Data: 24 calories | 0.7g carbs | 2.32g fat | 0.34g protein | 584mg sodium

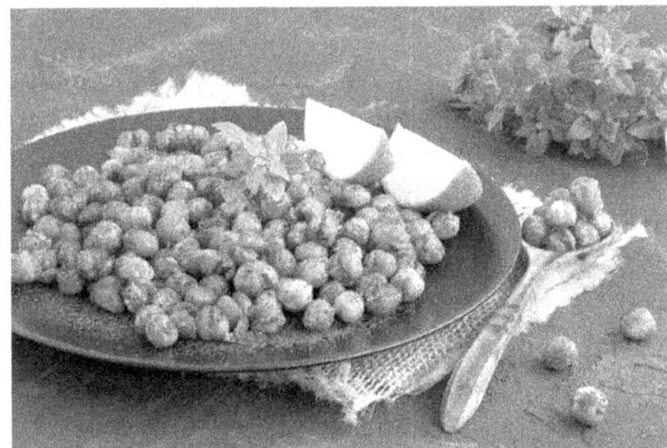

Preparation Time: 5 minutes
Cooking Time: 40 minutes
Serves: 12
Ingredients:

- 30-oz can chickpeas, drained, rinsed & patted dry
- 1/4 tsp cayenne
- 2 tbsp olive oil
- 3 tbsp hot sauce
- 2 tsp garlic powder
- 1 tbsp paprika

Directions:

Add chickpeas and remaining ingredients into mixing bowl and mix until well coated.

Spread chickpeas onto a parchment-lined baking sheet.

Roast chickpeas for 40 minutes at 425°F. Stir halfway through.

Serve and enjoy.

Nutritional Data: 122 calories | 16.98g carbs | 4.1g fat | 5.18g protein | 246mg sodium

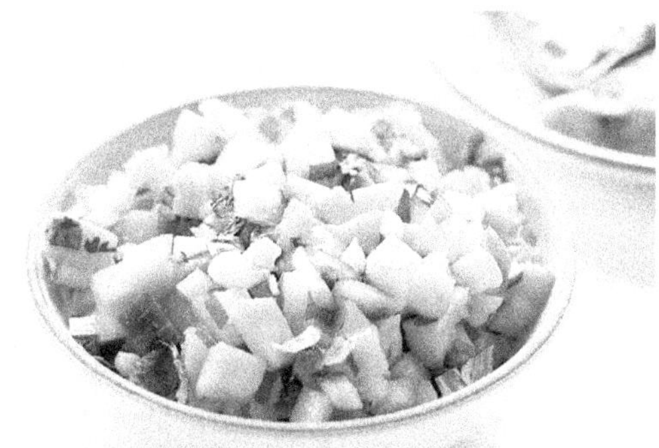

Preparation Time: 5 minutes
Cooking Time: 5 minutes
Serves: 4
Ingredients:

- 2 mangoes, peeled & diced
- 2 tbsp cilantro, chopped
- 1 jalapeno pepper, seeded & diced
- ½ lime juice
- ¼ cup onion, diced
- Pepper
- Salt

Directions:

In a bowl, mix together mango and remaining ingredients. Season salsa with pepper and salt.

Serve immediately and enjoy

Nutritional Data: 70 calories | 17.43g carbs | 0.43g fat | 1.19g protein | 3mg sodium

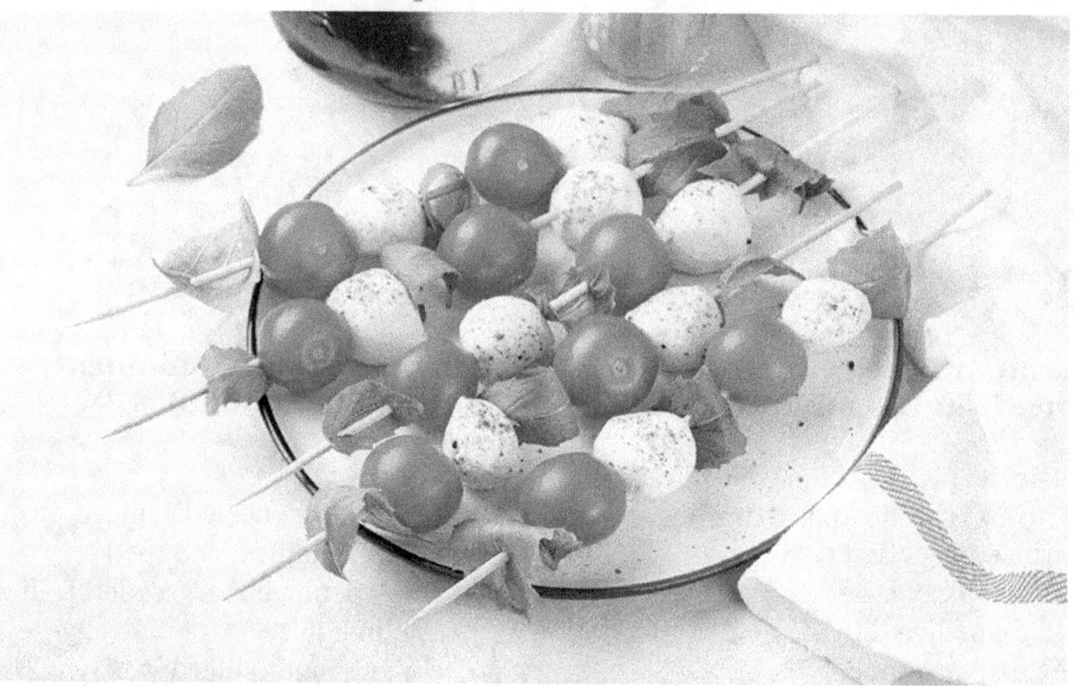

Preparation Time: 10 minutes
Cooking Time: 10 minutes
Serves: 12
Ingredients:

- 24 grape tomatoes
- 1 garlic clove, minced
- 12 mozzarella balls
- 24 basil leaves
- ½ tsp Italian seasoning
- 4 tbsp olive oil
- Pepper
- Salt

Directions:

In a bowl, mix together olive oil, garlic, Italian seasoning, mozzarella balls, pepper, and salt. Cover and place in refrigerator for 30 minutes to marinate.

Thread grape tomato on each skewer followed by a basil leaf, marinated mozzarella ball, another basil leave, and another tomato.

Serve and enjoy

Nutritional Data: 55 calories | 3.63g carbs | 4.57g fat | 0.34g protein | 14mg sodium

Chapter 4—Snack Recipes

1-Apple Slices with Almond Butter

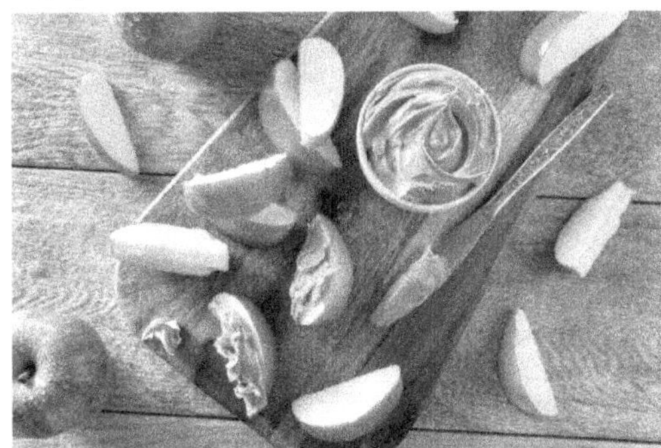

Preparation Time: 5 minutes
Cooking Time: 5 minutes
Serves: 2
Ingredients:

- 2 apples, cored & sliced
- ¼ cup almond butter
- ¼ cup cream cheese
- ½ tsp vanilla
- ¼ tsp cinnamon

Directions:

Add almond butter, cream cheese, vanilla, and cinnamon in a small bowl and beat using a hand mixer until fluffy.

Transfer almond butter to a serving bowl.

Serve with sliced apples.

Nutritional Data: 379 calories | 32.48g carbs | 26.24g fat | 9.17g protein | 204mg sodium

2-Trail Mix

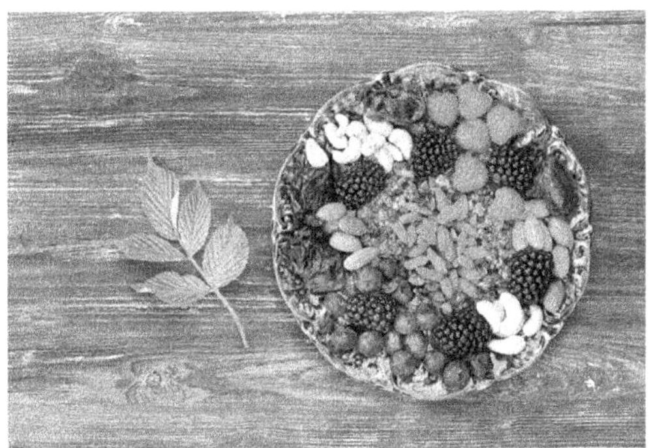

Preparation Time: 5 minutes
Cooking Time: 5 minutes
Serves: 6
Ingredients:

- 2 sections of dark chocolate, cut into small pieces
- 1/3 cup almond, sliced & toasted
- 1/3 cup cashews, roasted
- 2 tbsp dried cherries
- 2 tbsp dried cranberries
- ½ cup mulberries
- ½ cup goji berries

Directions:

Add all ingredients in a medium bowl and mix well.

Serve and enjoy.

Nutritional Data: 168 calories | 14.58g carbs | 11.56g fat | 2.93g protein | 47mg sodium

3-Greek Yogurt with Berries

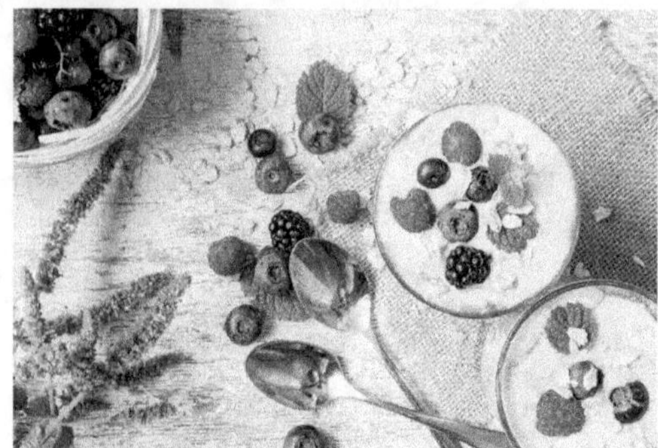

Preparation Time: 5 minutes
Cooking Time: 5 minutes
Serves: 1
Ingredients:

- ¾ cup Greek yogurt
- 1 tbsp almonds, sliced
- 2 mint leaves
- 1 tbsp honey
- ¼ cup raspberries
- ¼ cup blueberries
- ¼ cup strawberries, sliced

Directions:

Add Greek yogurt to serving bowl and top with berries.

Drizzle with honey and sprinkle with almond slices.

Garnish with mint leaves and serve.

Nutritional Data: 306 calories | 56.1g carbs | 1.73g fat | 20.35g protein | 71mg sodium

4-Carrot Sticks with Hummus

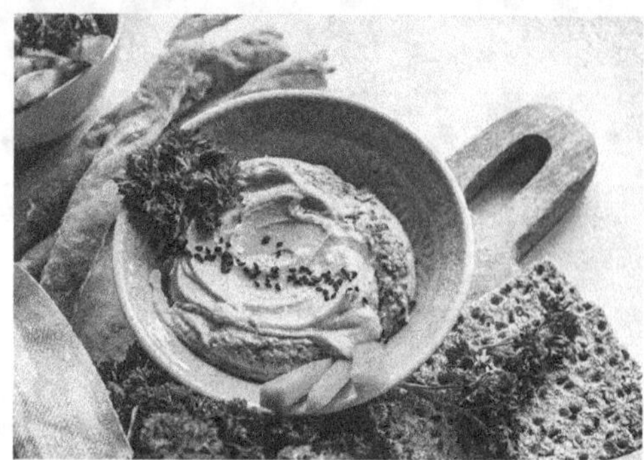

Preparation Time: 10 minutes
Cooking Time: 25 minutes
Serves: 4
Ingredients:

- 1 cup dry chickpeas, soaked overnight & drained
- 1/2 cup olive oil
- 1 tsp ground cumin
- 2 green chilies
- 1/2 cup fresh parsley
- 1 tbsp tahini
- 4 garlic cloves
- Pepper
- Salt
- 2 medium carrots, peeled & cut into small spears

Directions:

Add chickpeas into instant pot and cover with water.

Cover and cook on high pressure for 25 minutes.

Allow to release pressure naturally. Remove lid.

Drain chickpeas and transfer them into food processor.

Add remaining ingredients and process until smooth.

Transfer hummus to a serving bowl and serve with carrot sticks.

Nutritional Data: 387 calories | 18.12g carbs | 33.82g fat | 5.36g protein | 135mg sodium

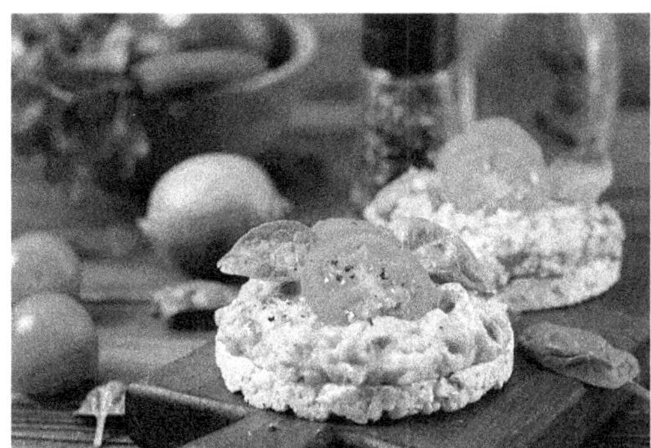

Preparation Time: 10 minutes
Cooking Time: 5 minutes
Serves: 2
Ingredients:

- 2 rice cakes
- 1 avocado, flesh scooped out
- 3 tbsp agave nectar
- ½ lime zest, grated
- 1 lime juice
- ¼ tsp salt

Directions:

Add avocado flesh into bowl and mash using a fork.

Add agave nectar, lime zest, lime juice, and salt and mix until well combined. Cover and place in refrigerator for 1 hour.

Spread avocado mixture on top of each rice cake and serve.

Nutritional Data: 209 calories | 19.66g carbs | 15.15g fat | 2.82g protein | 306mg sodium

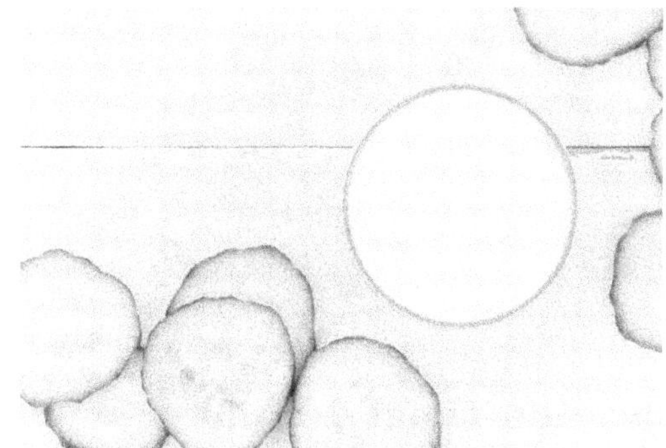

Preparation Time: 5 minutes
Cooking Time: 5 minutes
Serves: 6
Ingredients:

- 2 cups cottage cheese
- ¼ tsp red pepper flakes, crushed
- 1 tbsp olive oil
- 2 cucumbers, cut into slices

Directions:

Add cottage cheese to food processor and process until smooth.

Transfer cottage cheese to a serving bowl. Sprinkle with crushed red pepper flakes and drizzle with olive oil.

Serve with cucumber slices.

Nutritional Data: 90 calories | 2.59g carbs | 5.27g fat | 7.84g protein | 255mg sodium

7-Mixed Nuts

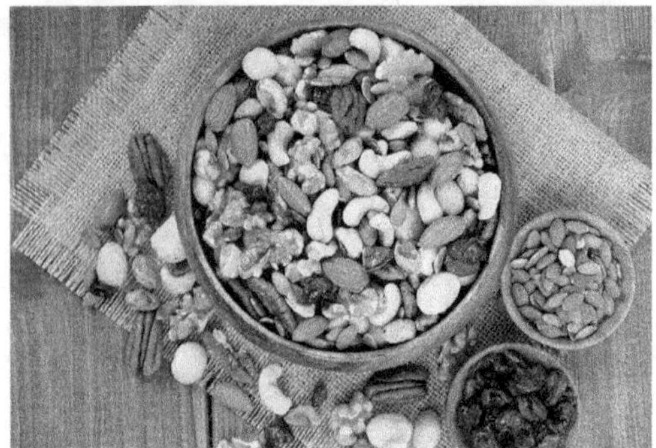

Preparation Time: 5 minutes
Cooking Time: 4 minutes
Serves: 6
Ingredients:

- 2 cups mixed nuts
- 1/4 tsp cayenne
- 1 tbsp olive oil
- 1 tsp ground cumin
- 1 tsp pepper
- 1 tsp salt

Directions:

In a bowl, add nuts and remaining ingredients and toss well.

Add the nuts mixture to the air fryer basket and air-fry for 4 minutes at 350°F.

Serve and enjoy.

Nutritional Data: 345 calories | 7.08g carbs | 36.2g fat | 3.76g protein | 391mg sodium

8-Chia Seed Pudding

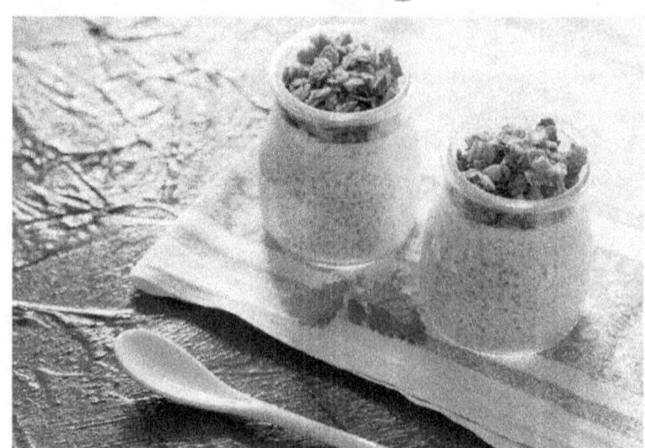

Preparation Time: 5 minutes
Cooking Time: 5 minutes
Serves: 4
Ingredients:

- ½ cup chia seeds
- 2 cups full-fat coconut milk
- 2 tbsp unsweetened shredded coconut
- 1 tsp turmeric
- 1 tsp cinnamon
- 3 tbsp maple syrup
- ¼ cup unsweetened almond milk

Directions:

In a medium bowl, whisk together coconut milk, turmeric, cinnamon, maple syrup, chia seeds, and almond milk. Cover and place in refrigerator for 2 hours.

Top with shredded coconut and serve.

Nutritional Data: 425 calories | 27.84g carbs | 35g fat | 6.31g protein | 42mg sodium

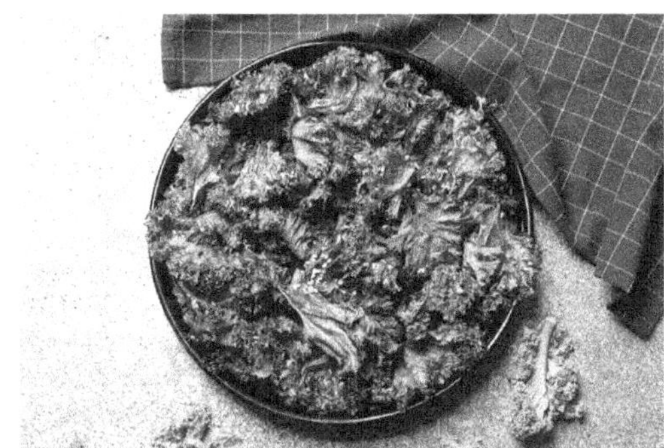

Preparation Time: 5 minutes
Cooking Time: 3 minutes
Serves: 2
Ingredients:

- 1 head kale, torn into 1 ½-inch pieces
- 1 tsp low-sodium soy sauce
- 1 tbsp olive oil

Directions:

Preheat air fryer to 400°F.

Add kale in a bowl and toss with soy sauce and oil.

Add kale into the air fryer basket and air-fry for 3 minutes.

Serve and enjoy.

Nutritional Data: 71 calories | 1.36g carbs | 7.31g fat | 0.53g protein | 43mg sodium

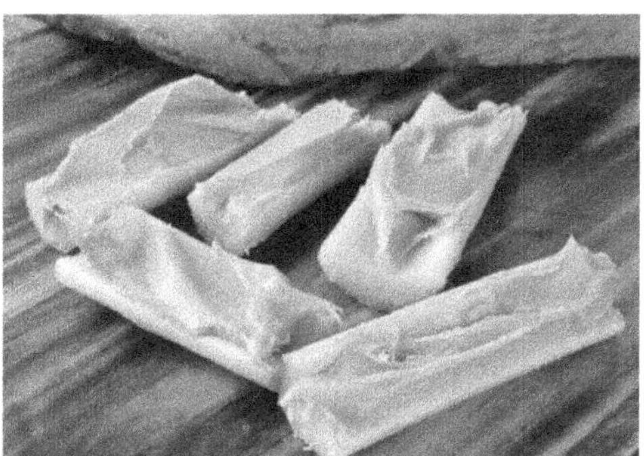

Preparation Time: 5 minutes
Cooking Time: 5 minutes
Serves: 1
Ingredients:

- 1 tbsp peanut butter, smooth
- 3 celery stalks, sliced
- Smoked paprika

Directions:

Cut celery stalks into 3-inch pieces.

Spread peanut butter to the center of each celery stalk and sprinkle with a pinch of smoked paprika.

Serve and enjoy.

Nutritional Data: 54 calories | 5.48g carbs | 2.97g fat | 1.49g protein | 282mg sodium

11-Edamame

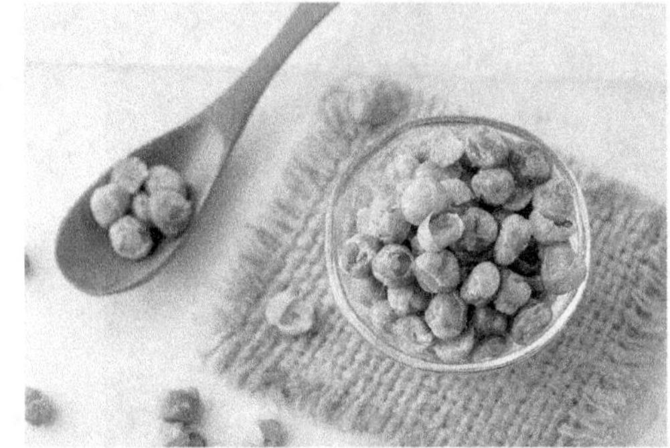

Preparation Time: 5 minutes
Cooking Time: 10 minutes
Serves: 4
Ingredients:

- 10 oz frozen edamame, shelled
- 1/4 tsp paprika
- 2 tbsp olive oil
- Pepper
- Salt

Directions:

In a bowl, toss edamame with paprika, oil, pepper, and salt.

Add edamame into air fryer basket and cook at 400°F for 10 minutes. Stir halfway through.

Serve and enjoy.

Nutritional Data: 151 calories | 8.19g carbs | 10.48g fat | 7.96g protein | 5mg sodium

12-Roasted Chickpeas

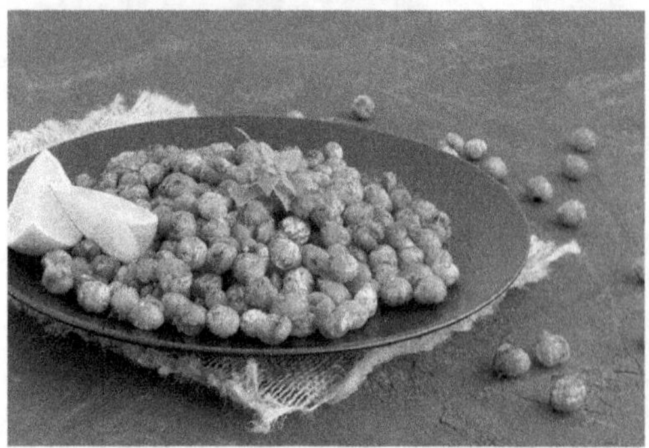

Preparation Time: 5 minutes
Cooking Time: 30 minutes
Serves: 4
Ingredients:

- 14.5-oz can chickpeas, rinsed & patted dry
- 1/2 tsp ground cumin
- 1/2 tsp paprika
- 1 tbsp olive oil
- Pepper
- Salt

Directions:

Preheat oven to 425°F.

Line baking sheet with parchment paper and set aside.

In a bowl, toss chickpeas with cumin, oil, paprika, pepper, and salt.

Spread chickpeas onto the baking sheet and bake for 30 minutes. Stir halfway through.

Serve and enjoy.

Nutritional Data: 179 calories | 24.5g carbs | 6.34g fat | 7.56g protein | 254mg sodium

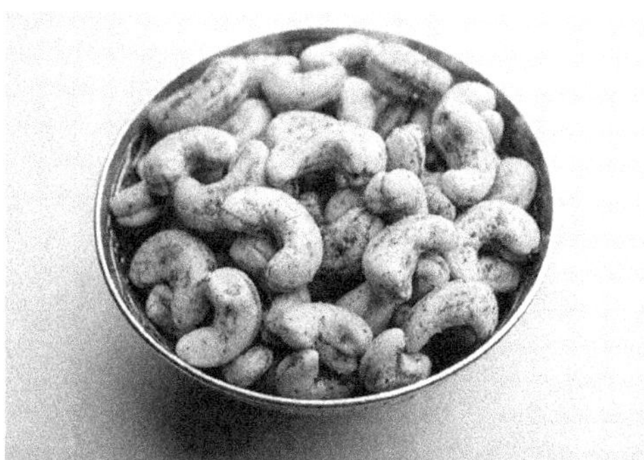

Preparation Time: 5 minutes
Cooking Time: 18 minutes
Serves: 10
Ingredients:
- 2 cups cashews
- 1 tsp garlic powder
- 2 tbsp date syrup
- ¼ cup sesame seeds
- ¼ cup dried seaweed
- 3 tbsp olive oil
- 1 tsp salt

Directions:

Preheat oven to 350°F.

Line baking sheet with parchment paper and set aside.

Spread cashews onto the baking sheet and bake for 8–10 minutes.

In a mixing bowl, mix together garlic powder, date syrup, sesame seeds, seaweed, olive oil, and salt. Add cashews and mix until well coated.

Spread cashews on a baking sheet and bake for 8 minutes more. Remove from oven and allow to cool completely.

Serve and enjoy.

Nutritional Data: 385 calories | 1969g carbs | 33.51g fat | 7.03g protein | 389mg sodium

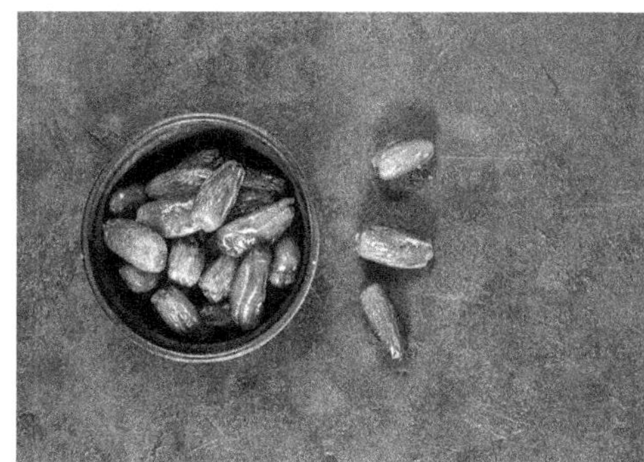

Preparation Time: 5 minutes
Cooking Time: 5 minutes
Serves: 2
Ingredients:
- 4 dates, pitted
- ½ tsp orange zest, grated
- 4 almonds, salted

Directions:

Stuff each date with a salted almond and roll in grated orange zest.

Serve and enjoy.

Nutritional Data: 55 calories | 11.32g carbs | 1.26g fat | 0.86g protein | 0mg sodium

15-Frozen Grapes

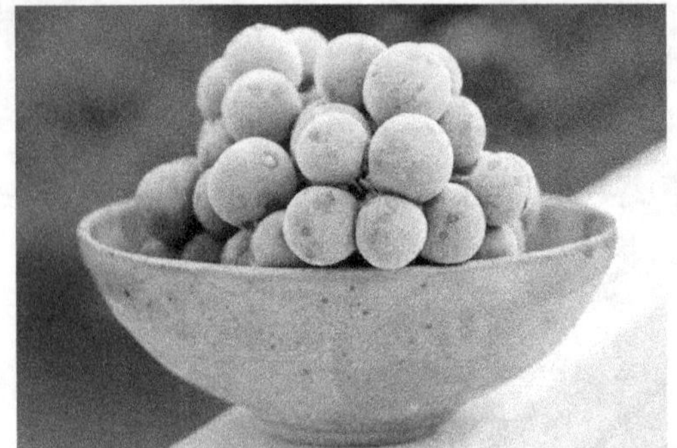

Preparation Time: 5 minutes
Cooking Time: 5 minutes
Serves: 2
Ingredients:

- 3 cups red grapes

Directions:

Add grapes in a colander and rinse well to remove pesticides and bacteria.

Gently pull the grapes from the stem.

Add grapes into zip-lock bag and place in the freezer for 6 hours.

Serve and enjoy.

Nutritional Data: 156 calories | 41g carbs | 0.36g fat | 1.63g protein | 5mg sodium

16-Coconut Yogurt Parfait

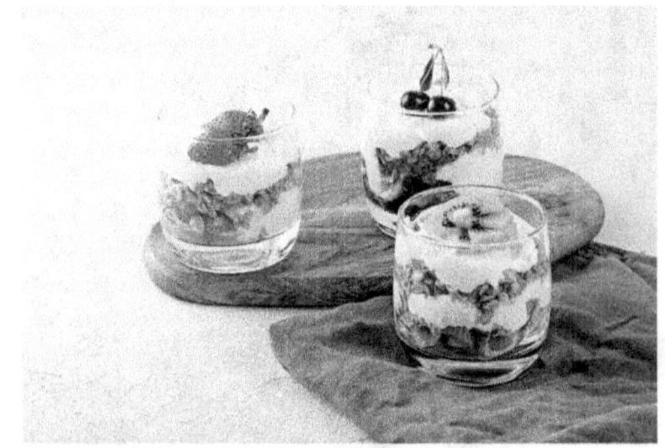

Preparation Time: 5 minutes
Cooking Time: 5 minutes
Serves: 2
Ingredients:

- 2 cups coconut yogurt
- 1 cup granola
- 1 cup fresh fruit, chopped

Directions:

Add ½ coconut yogurt to the bottom of two serving jars.

Top with 1/2 fruit, ½ granola, and repeat.

Serve immediately and enjoy.

Nutritional Data: 136 calories | 32.35g carbs | 0.57g fat | 2.21g protein | 259mg sodium

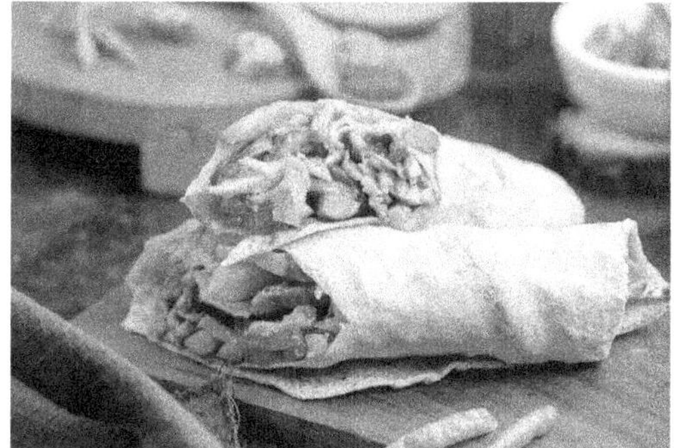

Preparation Time: 10 minutes
Cooking Time: 10 minutes
Serves: 12
Ingredients:
- 4 tortillas
- 8 Swiss cheese slices
- 8 deli turkey
- 8 lettuce leaves
- 2 green onions, chopped
- ½ cup sun-dried tomatoes, chopped
- 8 oz cream cheese, softened

Directions:

In a small bowl, mix together cream cheese, sun-dried tomatoes, and green onions.

Place a tortilla on a board and spread some cream cheese mixture on top of the tortilla.

Place two lettuce leaves in the center of the tortilla then place two cheese slices and top with two turkey slices.

Roll up the tortilla tightly and wrap it in plastic wrap. Place in the refrigerator until ready to serve.

Cut into slices and serve.

Nutritional Data: 247 calories | 24.68g carbs | 12.31g fat | 12.45g protein | 825mg sodium

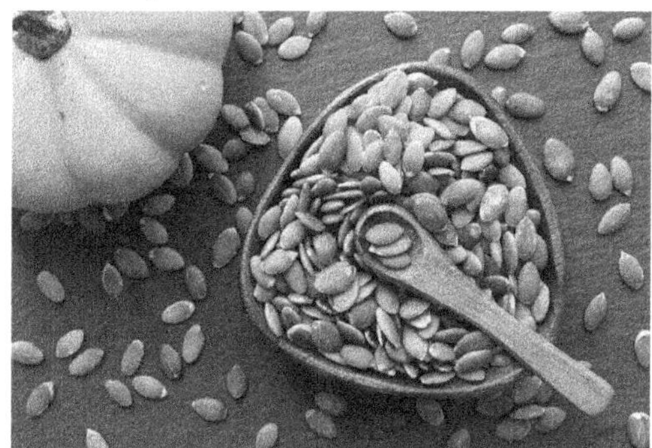

Preparation Time: 5 minutes
Cooking Time: 15 minutes
Serves: 4
Ingredients:
- 1 cup pumpkin seeds
- ¼ tsp garlic powder
- 1 tsp butter, melted
- ¼ tsp paprika
- 1/8 tsp pepper
- ¼ tsp salt

Directions:

Preheat air fryer to 360°F.

In a bowl, toss pumpkin seeds with paprika, butter, garlic, pepper, and salt.

Add pumpkin seeds into the air fryer basket and cook for 12–15 minutes. Stir halfway through.

Serve and enjoy.

Nutritional Data: 179 calories | 4.71g carbs | 15.45g fat | 8.9g protein | 229mg sodium

19-Bell Pepper Slices with Guacamole

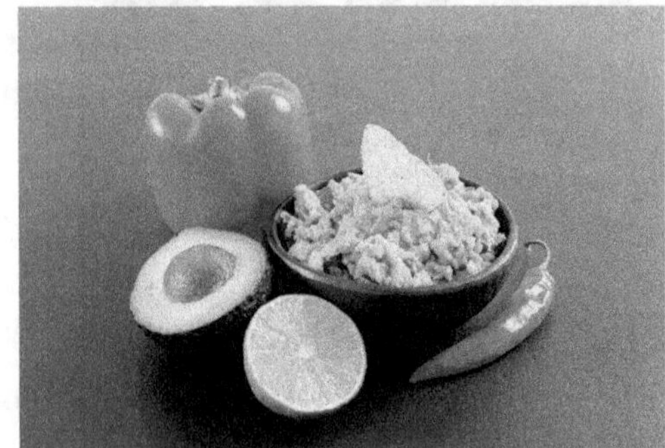

Preparation Time: 10 minutes
Cooking Time: 5 minutes
Serves: 4
Ingredients:

- 3 avocados, flesh scooped out
- 1 jalapeno, chopped
- 1/2 cup onion, chopped
- 2 tbsp lime juice
- 1/4 tsp hot sauce
- 4 tbsp cilantro, chopped
- 1/2 tbsp garlic, minced
- Pepper
- Salt
- 2 cups bell peppers, sliced

Directions:

Add avocado flesh into mixing bowl and mash using a fork.

Add remaining ingredients except bell pepper and mix well.

Serve with bell pepper slices.

Nutritional Data: 264 calories | 18.43g carbs | 22.2g fat | 3.97g protein | 22mg sodium

20-Apple Chips

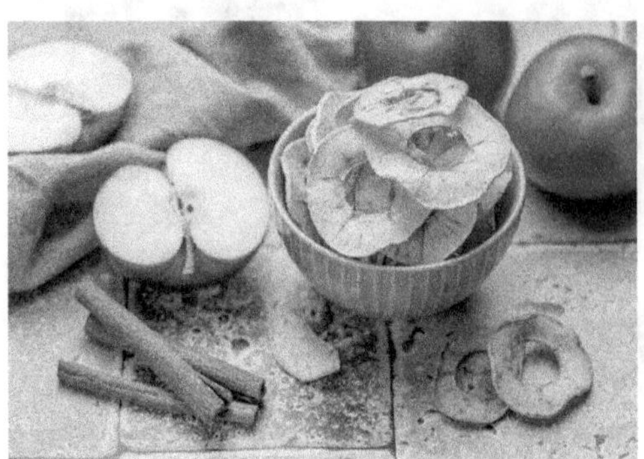

Preparation Time: 10 minutes
Cooking Time: 15 minutes
Serves: 2
Ingredients:

- 1 apple, thinly sliced
- 1/8 tsp ground cinnamon

Directions:

Arrange apple slices into air fryer basket and sprinkle with cinnamon.

Cook at 300°F for 15 minutes. Turn apple slices halfway through.

Serve and enjoy.

Nutritional Data: 48 calories | 12.69g carbs | 0.16g fat | 0.24g protein | 1mg sodium

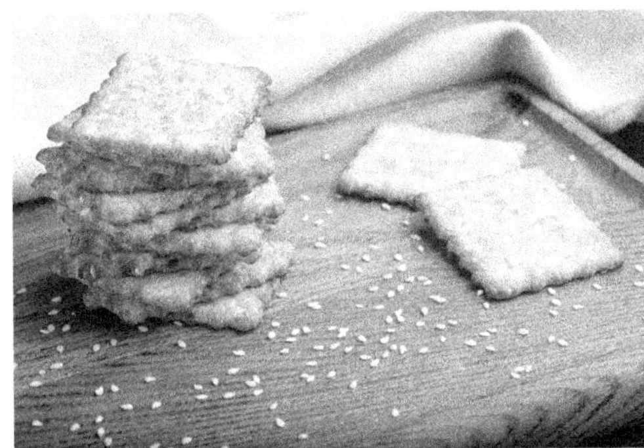

Preparation Time: 10 minutes
Cooking Time: 12 minutes
Serves: 6
Ingredients:
- 1 egg, lightly beaten
- 2 cups almond flour
- ½ tsp sea salt

Directions:

Preheat oven to 350°F.

Line baking sheet with parchment paper and set aside.

In a mixing bowl, add almond flour and salt and mix well. Add egg and mix until dough forms.

Divide dough between two cookie sheets and roll until 0.2 cm thick.

Cut into rectangle pieces and place on a parchment-lined baking sheet.

Bake in preheated oven for 8–12 minutes.

Serve and enjoy.

Nutritional Data: 24 calories | 0.26g carbs | 1.81g fat | 1.58g protein | 211mg sodium

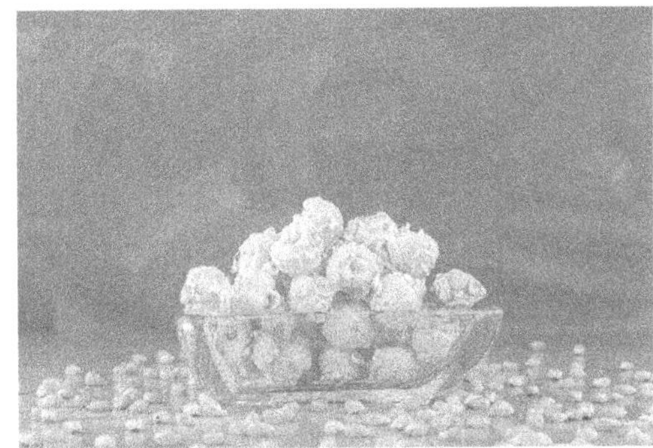

Preparation Time: 5 minutes
Cooking Time: 5 minutes
Serves: 6
Ingredients:
- ½ cup popcorn kernels
- 1 tbsp nutritional yeast
- ½ tsp ground turmeric
- 1 tsp curry powder
- 1 tbsp coconut oil
- ½ tsp sea salt

Directions:

Melt the coconut oil in a heavy saucepan.

Add popcorn kernels to melted oil and stir for a minute. Cover the pan with a lid to pop the popcorn.

Once popping slows down, remove the lid. Add curry powder, turmeric, nutritional yeast, and salt and mix well.

Serve and enjoy.

Nutritional Data: 103 calories | 13.93g carbs | 4.03g fat | 3.01g protein | 369mg sodium

23-Stuffed Mini Peppers

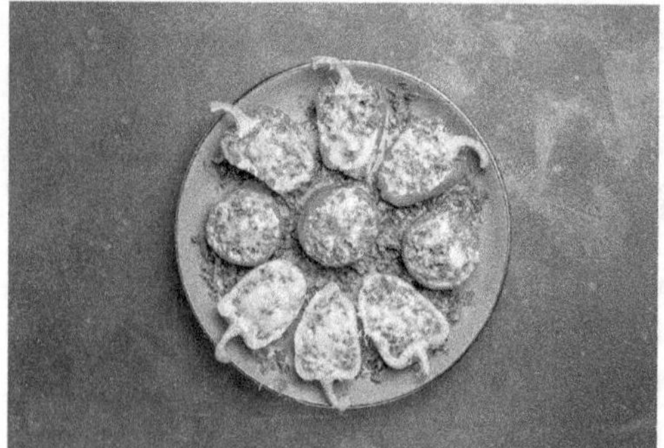

Preparation Time: 10 minutes
Cooking Time: 15 minutes
Serves: 8
Ingredients:

- 8 mini peppers, cut lengthwise & seeds removed
- 3 oz cooked chicken, shredded
- ½ tsp paprika
- ½ tsp garlic, minced
- 5 basil leaves, chopped
- 1 green onion, chopped
- 1 tbsp parsley, chopped
- 2 tbsp parmesan cheese, shredded
- ¼ cup cream cheese, softened
- Pepper
- Salt

Directions:

Preheat oven to 375°F.

In a mixing bowl, mix together shredded chicken, paprika, garlic, basil, green onion, parsley, parmesan cheese, cream cheese, pepper, and salt until well combined.

Stuff chicken mixture into each pepper and place onto a parchment-lined baking sheet.

Bake stuff peppers in preheated oven for 12–15 minutes.

Serve and enjoy.

Nutritional Data: 251 calories | 6.66g carbs | 22.7g fat | 8.33g protein | 65mg sodium

24-Anti-Inflammatory Smoothie

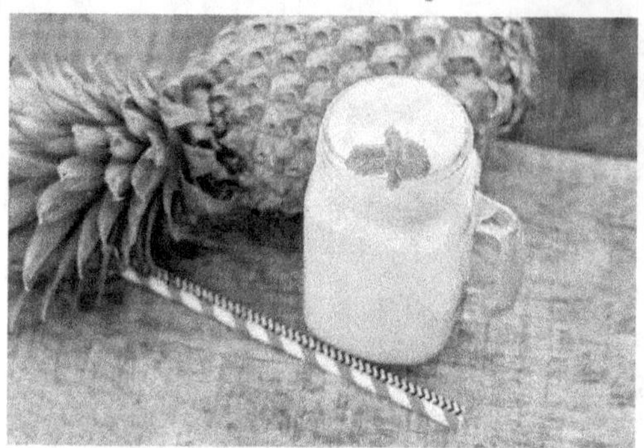

Preparation Time: 5 minutes
Cooking Time: 5 minutes
Serves: 2
Ingredients:

- 2 cups frozen pineapple chunks
- 1 tsp fresh ginger, grated
- 1 tbsp fresh turmeric, grated
- 1 banana
- 1 cup unsweetened almond milk

Directions:

Add pineapple chunks, ginger, turmeric, banana, and almond milk into blender and blend until smooth and creamy.

Serve immediately and enjoy.

Nutritional Data: 339 calories | 82.45g carbs | 2.1g fat | 2.85g protein | 92mg sodium

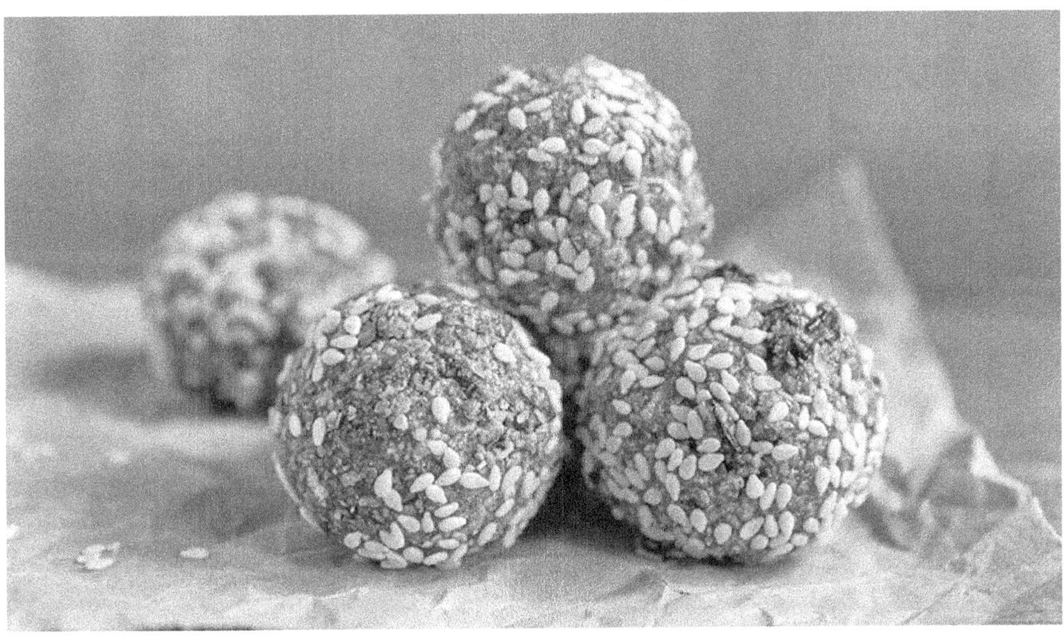

Preparation Time: 10 minutes
Cooking Time: 10 minutes
Serves: 12
Ingredients:

- ½ cup almond butter
- 2 tbsp dark chocolate chips
- 4 tbsp maple syrup
- 4 tbsp ground flaxseed
- ¾ cup shredded coconut
- ¾ cup oats
- Sea salt

Directions:

Add oats, ground flaxseed, shredded coconut, and salt into a mixing bowl and mix until combined.

Add chocolate, chips, maple syrup, and almond butter and mix well.

Make equal shapes of balls from the oat mixture and place onto the parchment-lined plate. Place the plate in the freezer for 20 minutes to set.

Serve and enjoy.

Nutritional Data: 126 calories | 12.93g carbs | 8.13g fat | 4.01g protein | 49mg sodium

Chapter 5—Lunch Recipes

1-Salmon Salad

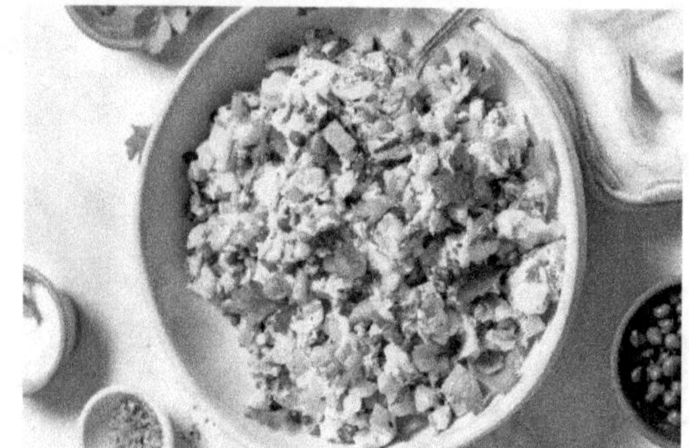

Preparation Time: 10 minutes
Cooking Time: 20 minutes
Serves: 2
Ingredients:

- 8 oz salmon, cooked
- 1 small onion, chopped
- 2 tbsp cilantro, chopped
- 1 cup sweet potatoes, roasted & chopped
- ½ cup radishes, chopped
- 2 cups lettuce, chopped
- 1 cup arugula
- 1 cucumber, chopped
- 1 tbsp olive oil
- 1 tsp garlic, minced
- 2 tbsp ginger, grated
- 1 lemon, juiced
- ½ avocado, chopped
- Pepper
- Salt

Directions:

In a bowl, toss sweet potatoes with oil and season with pepper and salt.

Spread sweet potatoes onto a baking sheet and bake for 20 minutes at 400°F or until cooked.

Add salmon into the large mixing bowl and flake the salmon using a fork.

Add roasted sweet potatoes, onion, cilantro, radishes, lettuce, arugula, cucumber, olive oil, garlic, ginger, lemon juice, and avocado, and mix everything well. Season salad with pepper and salt.

Serve and enjoy.

Nutritional Data: 500 calories | 46.71g carbs | 23.05g fat | 29.58g protein | 562mg sodium

2-Quinoa Salad

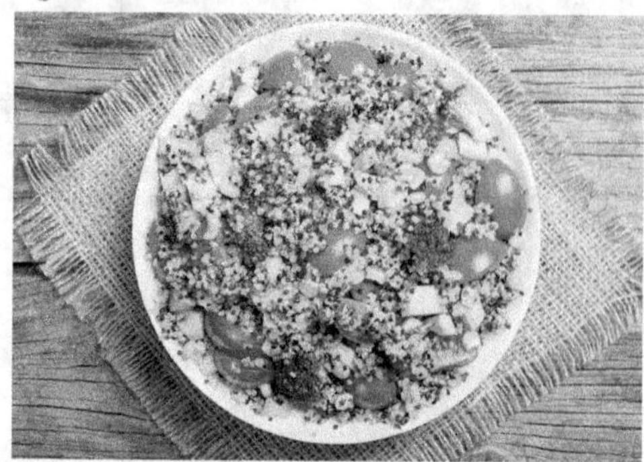

Preparation Time: 10 minutes
Cooking Time: 5 minutes
Serves: 4
Ingredients:

- 1 cup cooked quinoa
- 1 tbsp olive oil
- ½ lemon, juiced
- 1 tsp vinegar
- 8 basil leaves, chopped
- ½ cup parsley, chopped
- ½ cup arugula, chopped
- 1 avocado, diced
- ½ cup tomatoes, chopped
- 1 spring onion, chopped
- ½ cup olives, pitted & chopped
- 1 red bell pepper, chopped
- Salt

Directions:

Add cooked quinoa and remaining ingredients into large mixing bowl and mix everything well.

Cover salad bowl and place in refrigerator for 1 hour.

Serve and enjoy.

Nutritional Data: 199 calories | 18.27g carbs | 13.59g fat | 3.98g protein | 138mg sodium

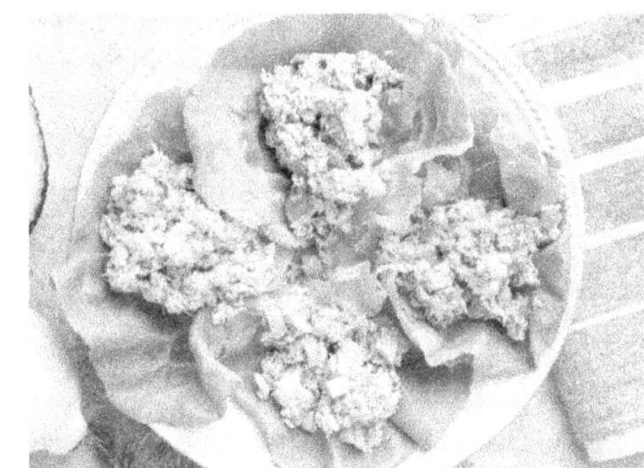

Preparation Time: 5 minutes
Cooking Time: 5 minutes
Serves: 8
Ingredients:

- 10-oz can tuna, drained
- 8 romaine lettuce leaves
- 2 green onions, sliced
- ½ cup carrots, chopped
- 2 celery ribs, diced
- For sauce:
- ½ cup cashews, soaked in water for 2 hours
- 1 garlic clove
- ½ cup water
- ¼ tsp salt

Directions:

Add cashews, garlic, water, and salt into blender and blend until smooth.

Add tuna into mixing bowl and break using a fork. Add green onions, carrots, celery, and cashew sauce and mix until well combined.

Divide the tuna mixture evenly onto the lettuce leaves and serve immediately.

Nutritional Data: 135 calories | 6.34g carbs | 8.89g fat | 9.09g protein | 222mg sodium

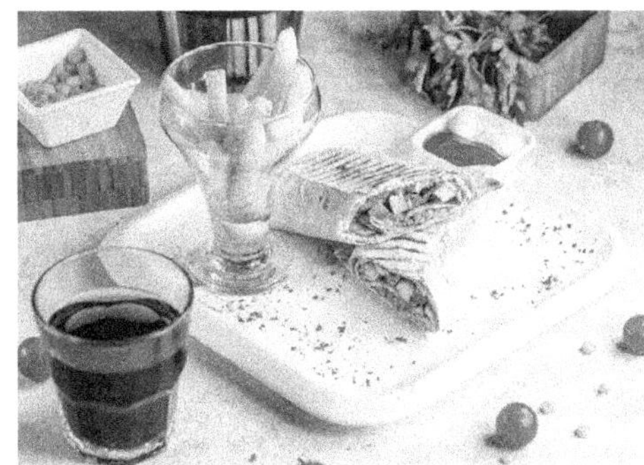

Preparation Time: 5 minutes
Cooking Time: 5 minutes
Serves: 1
Ingredients:

- 1 whole-wheat tortilla
- ¼ cup lettuce
- ¼ cup cucumber, sliced
- ¼ cup tomato, sliced
- ¼ cup avocado, sliced
- 2 cooked turkey bacon slices
- 2 oz deli turkey
- 1 tbsp Dijon mustard
- 1 tbsp mayonnaise

Directions:

Mix together mustard and mayonnaise and spread onto the tortilla.

Arrange deli turkey, turkey bacon slices, avocado, tomato, cucumber, and lettuce on the center of the tortilla.

Roll up the wrap tightly and cut it in half.

Serve and enjoy.

Nutritional Data: 692 calories | 34.31g carbs | 34.96g fat | 67.66g protein | 1835mg sodium

5-Vegetable Stir-Fry

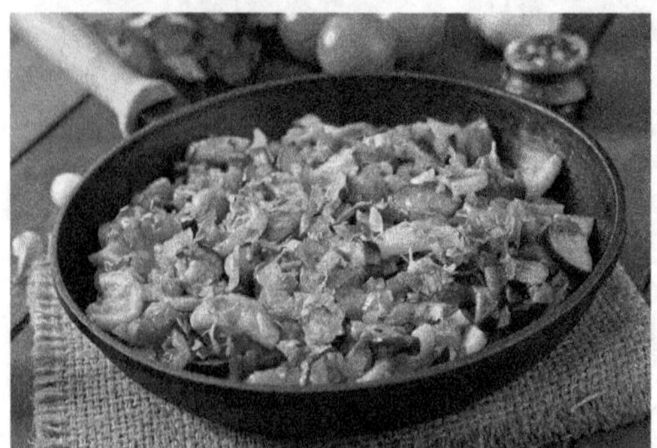

Preparation Time: 10 minutes
Cooking Time: 15 minutes
Serves: 4
Ingredients:

- 1 red bell pepper, seeded & sliced
- 8 oz mushrooms, sliced
- 8 oz can baby corn spears, drained
- 2 cups broccoli florets
- 1 carrot, peeled & sliced
- 2 tsp ginger, minced
- 1 tbsp garlic, minced
- 2 tbsp butter
- 2 tbsp olive oil
- ¼ tsp hot sauce
- 2 tbsp honey
- 3 tbsp low-sodium soy sauce
- ½ tsp cornstarch
- ¼ cup chicken broth

Directions:

Heat olive oil in a large pan over medium heat.

Add vegetables and stir-fry for 3 minutes. Add ginger, garlic, and butter, and cook for 1–2 minutes.

In a small bowl, mix together chicken broth, cornstarch, soy sauce, honey, and hot sauce and pour over vegetables. Cook over medium-low heat for 3–4 minutes or until sauce thickens.

Serve and enjoy.

Nutritional Data: 442 calories | 68.26g carbs | 16.58g fat | 14.35g protein | 542mg sodium

6-Sweet Potato-and-Black Bean Bowl

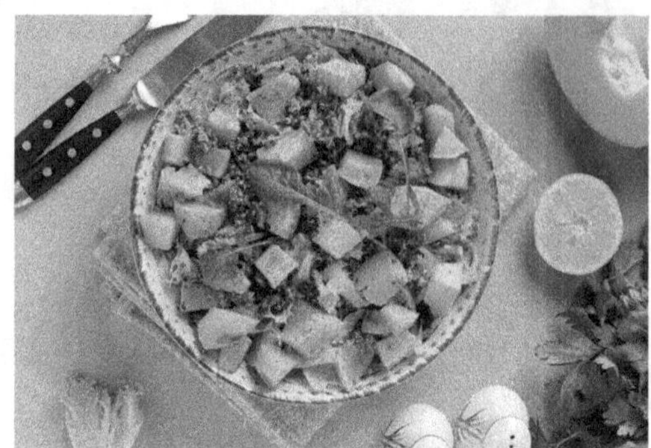

Preparation Time: 10 minutes
Cooking Time: 30 minutes
Serves: 4
Ingredients:

- 15.5-oz can black beans, drained & rinsed
- 2 medium sweet potatoes, cubed
- 1 cup guacamole
- 3 cups cooked brown rice
- ½ cup enchilada sauce
- 1 tbsp olive oil
- Pepper
- Salt

Directions:

Preheat oven to 425°F.

In a bowl, toss sweet potatoes with oil and season with pepper and salt.

Spread sweet potatoes onto a baking sheet and roast in preheated oven for 30 minutes.

In a small pot, add enchilada sauce and heat over medium heat. Add beans and cooked sweet potatoes and cook for 2 minutes. Remove from heat and set aside.

Divide the cooked brown rice into serving bowls and top with the enchilada mixture.

Top with guacamole and serve.

Nutritional Data: 946 calories | 171.57g carbs | 18.33g fat | 26.27g protein | 688mg sodium

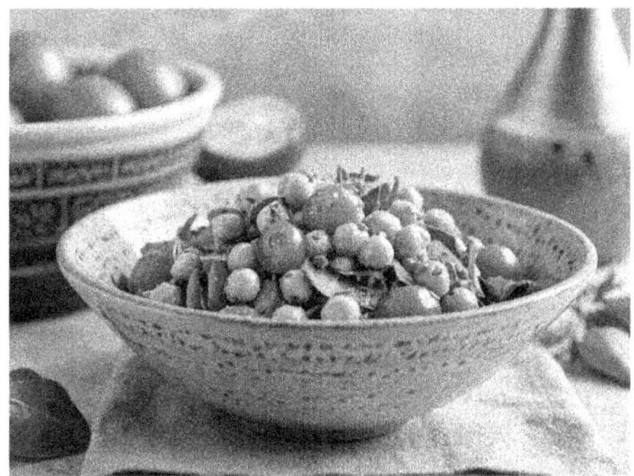

Preparation Time: 10 minutes
Cooking Time: 5 minutes
Serves: 8
Ingredients:

- 28-oz can chickpeas, drained & rinsed
- ¾ cup feta cheese, crumbled
- ¼ cup parsley, chopped
- 1/3 cup basil, chopped
- ½ cup onion, diced
- 1 red bell pepper, diced
- 2 cups cherry tomatoes, cut in half
- 1 cucumber, chopped
- For dressing:
- 1/3 cup olive oil
- 1 tbsp dried oregano
- ½ lemon, juiced
- 3 tbsp red wine vinegar
- ½ tsp pepper
- 1 tsp salt

Directions:

In a small bowl, whisk together all dressing ingredients and set aside.

In a mixing bowl, add chickpeas, crumbled cheese, parsley, basil, onion, bell pepper, cherry tomatoes, and cucumber. Mix well.

Pour dressing over salad and mix everything well. Cover salad and place in refrigerator for 30 minutes.

Serve and enjoy.

Nutritional Data: 266 calories | 25.98g carbs | 14.45g fat | 9.5g protein | 633mg sodium

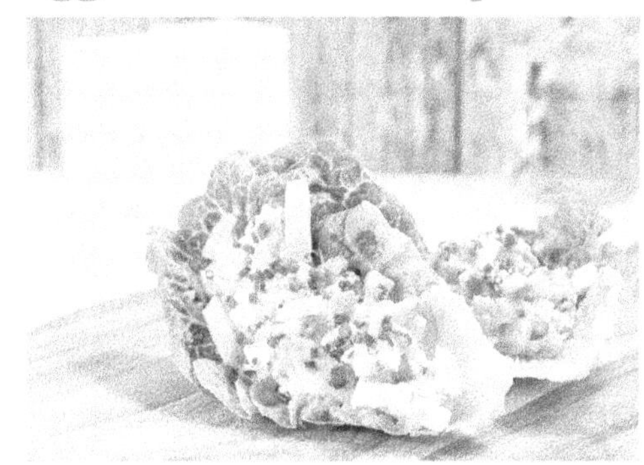

Preparation Time: 10 minutes
Cooking Time: 5 minutes
Serves: 2
Ingredients:

- 6 hard-boiled eggs, peeled & diced
- ¼ cup cilantro, chopped
- ¼ cup scallions, sliced
- 1 ½ tsp Dijon mustard
- ¼ tsp ground turmeric
- ½ cup Greek yogurt
- ¼ tsp sea salt

Directions:

In a mixing bowl, mix together yogurt, turmeric, mustard, and salt.

Add eggs, cilantro, and scallions, and mix everything well.

Serve salad on lettuce leaves.

Nutritional Data: 270 calories | 4.96g carbs | 16.28g fat | 24.42g protein | 539mg sodium

9-Cauliflower Rice Bowl

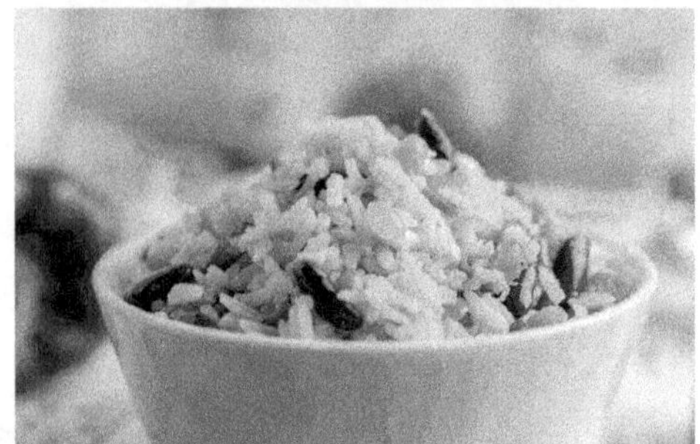

Preparation Time: 10 minutes
Cooking Time: 10 minutes
Serves: 6
Ingredients:

- 3 cups cauliflower rice
- ½ tsp cumin
- ½ tsp paprika
- 1 tsp chili powder
- ¼ cup salsa
- ¼ cup vegetable broth
- 1 can corn, rinsed & drained
- 1 can black beans, rinsed & drained
- 1 lb ground chicken
- 1 tbsp olive oil
- 2 garlic cloves, minced
- 1 small onion, diced
- Pepper
- Salt

Directions:

Heat olive oil in a large pan over medium-high heat.

Add onion and garlic and sauté until onion is softened.

Add ground chicken, cumin, paprika, chili powder, pepper, and salt, and cook until meat is cooked through.

Add corn, black beans, salsa, and cauliflower rice and stir well. Turn heat to low and cook for 8–10 minutes or until cauliflower is translucent.

Serve and enjoy.

Nutritional Data: 498 calories | 67.47g carbs | 21.65g fat | 30.07g protein | 373mg sodium

10-Chicken-and-Vegetable Soup

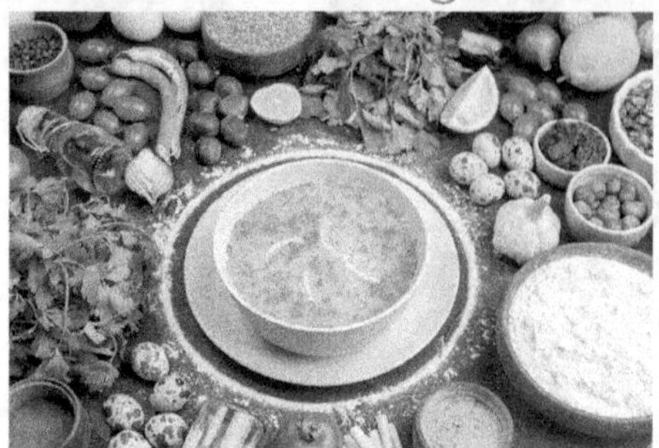

Preparation Time: 10 minutes
Cooking Time: 25 minutes
Serves: 4
Ingredients:

- 2 chicken breasts, boneless & skinless
- 2 cups fresh spinach, chopped
- 2 medium potatoes, cut into ½-inch pieces
- 14 oz-can tomatoes, diced
- 4 cups chicken broth
- 2 tsp Italian seasoning
- 1 tbsp garlic, minced
- ½ onion, diced
- 2 carrots, peeled & chopped
- 2 celery ribs, chopped
- 2 tbsp olive oil
- Pepper
- Salt

Directions:

Heat olive oil in a large pot over medium-high heat.

Add onion, carrots, and celery, and cook for 5–6 minutes.

Add Italian seasoning, garlic, pepper, and salt and cook for 1 minute.

Add broth, potatoes, chicken, and tomatoes. Stir well and bring to simmer over high heat. Turn heat to medium-low and simmer for 15 minutes or until chicken is cooked through.

Remove chicken from pot and shred using a fork.

Return shredded chicken to the pot along with spinach and stir well. Season with pepper and salt.

Serve and enjoy.

Nutritional Data: 942 calories | 44.86g carbs | 40.16g fat | 96.54g protein | 1361mg sodium

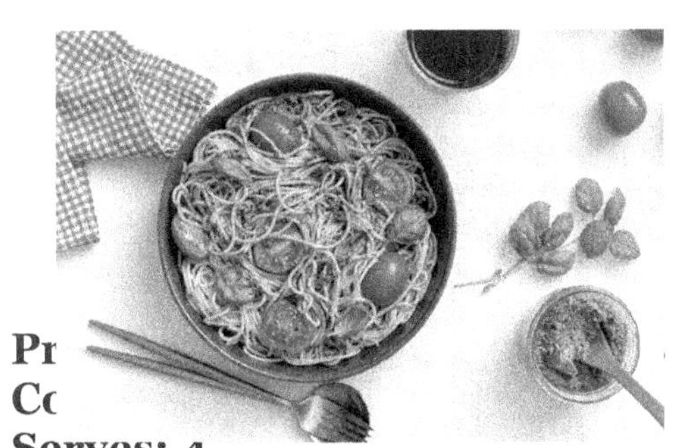

Pr
Co
Serves: 4
Ingredients:

- For pesto:
- 2 cups basil leaves
- ½ cup parmesan cheese, grated
- 2/3 cup olive oil
- ¼ cup pine nuts
- 2 garlic cloves
- Pepper
- Salt
- For zoodles:
- 4 zucchinis, spiralized
- 8 oz mozzarella pearls
- 2 cups grape tomatoes, halved
- 1 tbsp olive oil
- ¼ tsp salt

Directions:

Add all pesto ingredients into blender and blend until smooth.

In a mixing bowl, mix together zucchini noodles, mozzarella pearls, grape tomatoes, olive oil, pesto, and salt until well coated.

Serve immediately and enjoy.

Nutritional Data: 720 calories | 62.49g carbs | 49.66g fat | 11.5g protein | 380mg sodium

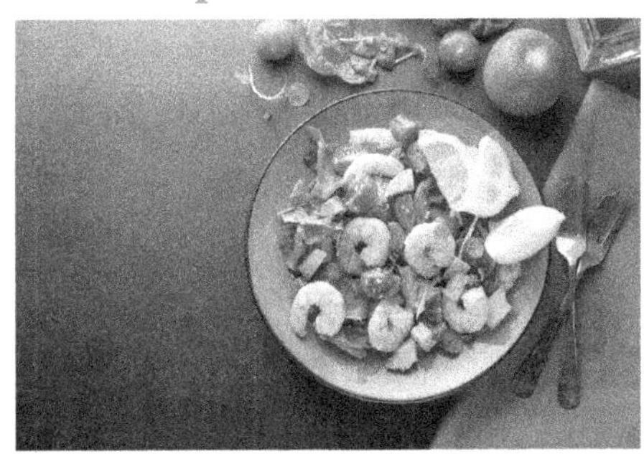

Preparation Time: 10 minutes
Cooking Time: 8 minutes
Serves: 2
Ingredients:

- ¾ lb shrimp, peeled & deveined
- 2 tsp mustard
- 3 tbsp mayonnaise
- ½ cup dill
- ½ onion, diced
- 1 tomato, chopped
- ½ avocado, sliced
- 3 celery sticks, chopped
- ½ tsp Cajun seasoning
- 1 tbsp olive oil
- ¼ tsp paprika
- 1 tbsp lemon juice
- Pepper
- Salt

Directions:

Season shrimp with Cajun seasoning, olive oil, paprika, pepper, and salt.

Add shrimp into air fryer basket and cook at 400°F for 8 minutes.

In a mixing bowl, add cooked shrimp, mustard, mayonnaise, dill, onion, tomato, avocado, and celery and mix well.

Serve and enjoy.

Nutritional Data: 447 calories | 18.11g carbs | 24.29g fat | 39.78g protein | 1892mg sodium

13-Lentil Salad

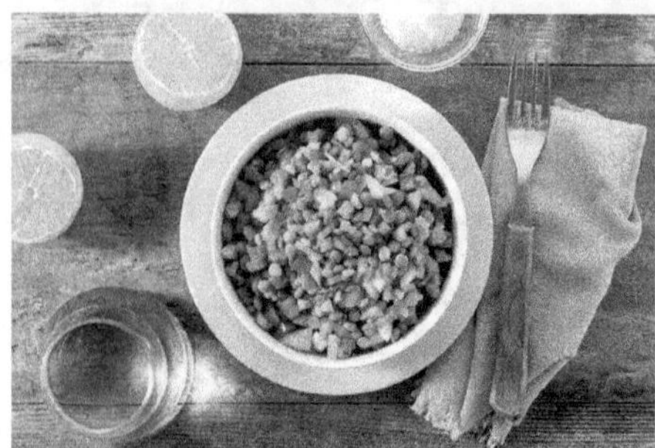

Preparation Time: 10 minutes
Cooking Time: 5 minutes
Serves: 6
Ingredients:

- 3 cups cooked brown lentils
- ½ cup onion, chopped
- 1 cup cucumber, diced
- 1 red bell pepper, diced
- 1 cup feta cheese, crumbled
- 1/3 cup olive oil
- 2 tsp Dijon mustard
- 1/3 cup dill, chopped
- 1/3 cup fresh lemon juice
- Pepper
- Salt

Directions:

Add cooked lentils and remaining ingredients into large mixing bowl and mix everything well.

Serve and enjoy.

Nutritional Data: 149 calories | 6.04g carbs | 8.1g fat | 13.26g protein | 631mg sodium

14-Stuffed Bell Peppers

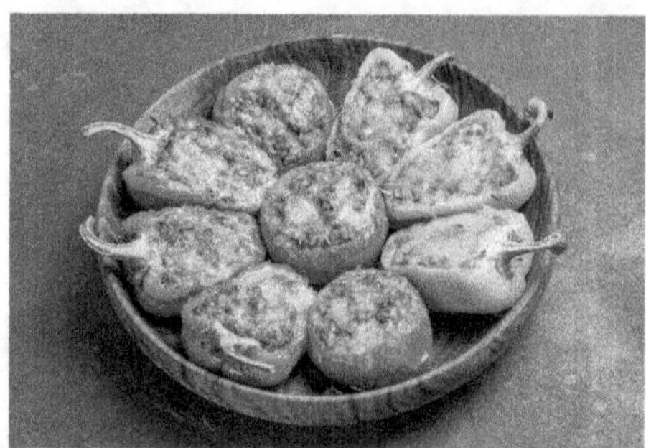

Preparation Time: 10 minutes
Cooking Time: 20 minutes
Serves: 6
Ingredients:

- 3 bell peppers, cut in half lengthwise & seeds removed
- 1 tbsp olive oil
- 1 lemon, juiced
- 1 /4 cup basil leaves, chopped
- 1 tbsp garlic, minced
- 2 cups cherry tomatoes, halved
- 2 cups cooked quinoa
- 1 lb cooked chicken breast, chopped
- Pepper
- Salt

Directions:

Preheat oven to 375°F.

In a mixing bowl, mix together chicken, quinoa, cherry tomatoes, garlic, basil, lemon juice, olive oil, pepper, and salt until well combined.

Stuff the chicken-quinoa mixture into each pepper half and place onto a baking sheet.

Bake in preheated oven for 20 minutes.

Serve and enjoy.

Nutritional Data: 632 calories | 27.26g carbs | 43.81g fat | 38.46g protein | 62mg sodium

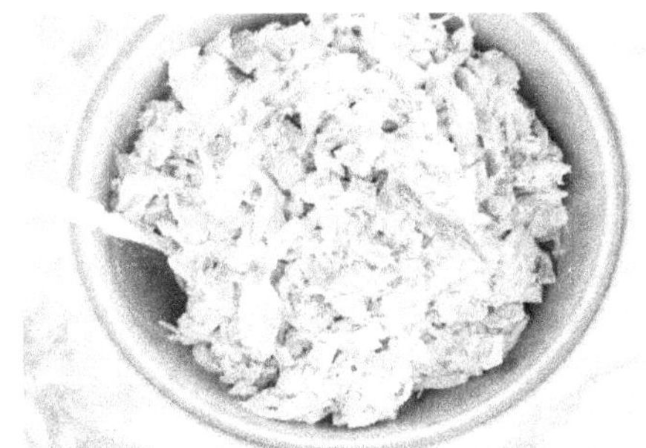

Preparation Time: 10 minutes
Cooking Time: 5 minutes
Serves: 4
Ingredients:

- 2 cooked chicken breasts, cut into cubes
- 2 tbsp fresh cilantro, chopped
- ½ cup raisins
- ½ cup cashews, roasted & chopped
- ¼ cup onion, diced
- 2 carrots, chopped
- ½ cup celery, chopped
- For dressing:
- ½ cup Greek yogurt
- 2 tbsp lime juice
- 1 tbsp honey
- 2 tbsp curry powder
- 3 tbsp mayonnaise
- ¼ tsp pepper
- ½ tsp kosher salt

Directions:

In a mixing bowl, mix together chicken, cilantro, raisins, cashews, onion, carrots, and celery.

In a small bowl, whisk together all dressing ingredients until smooth.

Pour dressing over salad and toss well.

Serve and enjoy.

Nutritional Data: 435 calories | 21.98g carbs | 24.27g fat | 34.79g protein | 579mg sodium

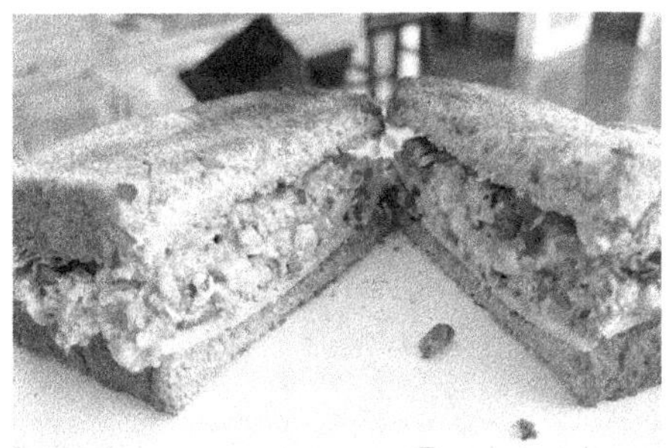

Preparation Time: 10 minutes
Cooking Time: 5 minutes
Serves: 2
Ingredients:

- 8.46-oz can sardines, drained
- 4 whole-grain bread slices, toasted
- 2 tbsp parsley, chopped
- 1 tbsp fresh lemon juice
- 1 lemon, zested
- 1 tbsp capers, drained
- 1 celery rib, diced
- ¼ cup scallions, thinly sliced
- 1 tbsp ground mustard
- 1 tbsp mayonnaise

Directions:

Add sardines into mixing bowl and mash using a fork. Add parsley, lemon juice, lemon zest, capers, celery, scallions, mustard, and mayonnaise and mix until well combined.

Spread the sardine mixture on one side of the bread slice then top with another bread slice. Assemble the remaining sandwich.

Serve and enjoy.

Nutritional Data: 561 calories | 39.88g carbs | 24.31g fat | 44.92g protein | 920mg sodium

17-Spinach-and-Strawberry Salad

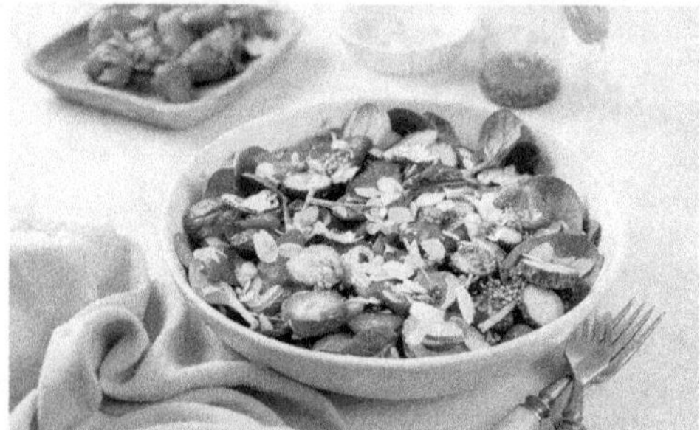

Preparation Time: 10 minutes
Cooking Time: 5 minutes
Serves: 6
Ingredients:

- 5 oz baby spinach, rinsed & patted dry
- ½ cup vinaigrette
- ½ cup feta cheese, crumbled
- 2 avocados, diced
- 1 cup blueberries, rinsed
- 4 cups strawberries, rinsed & halved
- ½ cup pecans, toasted & chopped

Directions:

In a mixing bowl, mix together spinach, crumbled cheese, avocados, blueberries, strawberries, and pecans.

Pour vinaigrette over the salad and toss well.

Serve immediately and enjoy.

Nutritional Data: 284 calories | 28.87g carbs | 19.87g fat | 5.5g protein | 385mg sodium

18-Tofu-and-Vegetable Stir-Fry

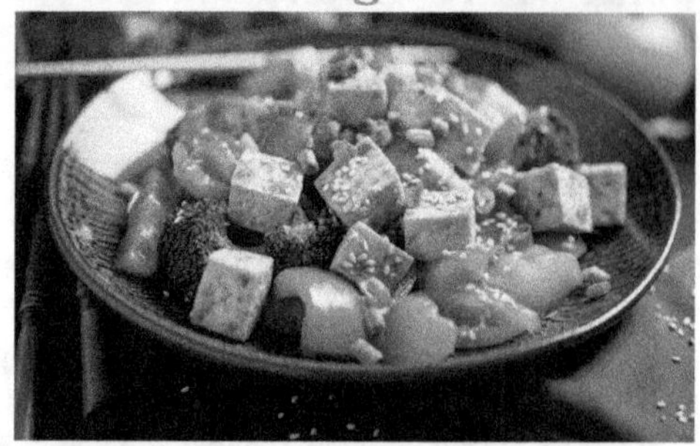

Preparation Time: 10 minutes
Cooking Time: 10 minutes
Serves: 4
Ingredients:

- 1 lb extra-firm tofu, cut into 1/2-inch chunks
- 1 tbsp rice vinegar
- 1 tsp red pepper flakes, crushed
- 2 tbsp rice wine
- ¼ cup low-sodium soy sauce
- 4 tbsp fermented black beans, rinsed
- 1 cup broccoli florets
- 1 cup mushrooms, halved
- 1 cup green beans
- 1 zucchini, sliced
- 1 carrot, thinly sliced
- 1 cup snow peas
- ½ cup baby corn, cut into ½-inch chunks
- 1 tsp garlic, minced
- 1 tbsp sesame oil
- ¼ cup olive oil

Directions:

Heat olive oil in a large pan over medium-high heat.

Add tofu and cook on all sides until seared and lightly golden brown.

Add broccoli, mushrooms, green beans, zucchini, carrots, snow peas, baby corn, and garlic and cook for 4–6 minutes.

In a small bowl, mix together sesame oil, vinegar, red pepper flakes, rice wine, soy sauce, and black beans and pour into the pan.

Stir well and cook for 3–4 minutes.

Serve and enjoy.

Nutritional Data: 451 calories | 35.3g carbs | 28.67g fat | 19.28g protein | 265mg sodium

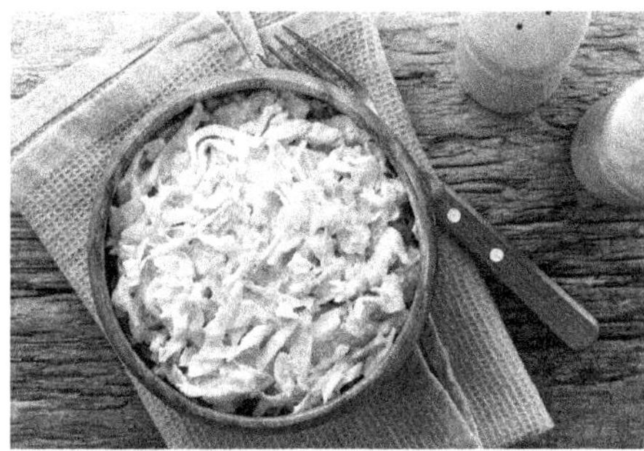

Preparation Time: 10 minutes
Cooking Time: 5 minutes
Serves: 6
Ingredients:

- 1 cabbage head, thinly sliced
- ½ cup almonds, sliced
- ½ cup fresh cilantro, chopped
- 2 green apples, cored & sliced into matchsticks
- For dressing:
- 1/3 cup vegan mayonnaise
- 1 tbsp honey
- 2 tbsp fresh lemon juice
- Pepper
- Salt

Directions:

In a small bowl, whisk together all dressing ingredients and set aside.

In a large bowl, mix cabbage, almonds, cilantro, and apples. Add dressing and toss well to combine.

Serve and enjoy.

Nutritional Data: 301 calories | 23.53g carbs | 19.11g fat | 12.85g protein | 177mg sodium

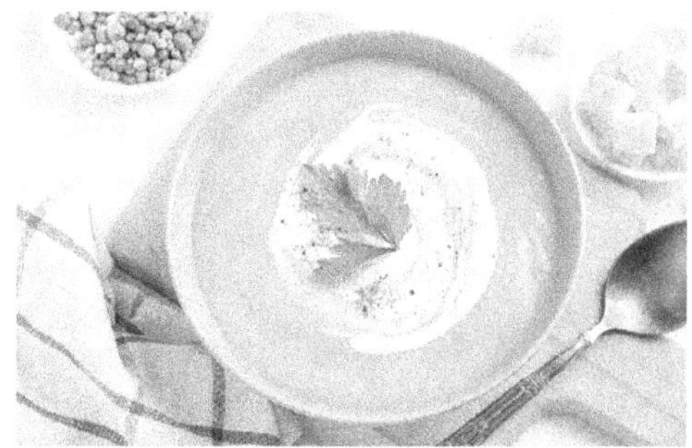

Preparation Time: 10 minutes
Cooking Time: 40 minutes
Serves: 4
Ingredients:

- 1 cup butternut squash, chopped
- 14.5 oz coconut milk
- 3 cups vegetable broth
- 1 tbsp turmeric powder
- 1 tbsp ginger, grated
- 2 garlic cloves, minced
- 3 cups carrots, chopped
- 1 cup fennel, chopped
- 1 leek, cleaned & sliced
- 1 tbsp olive oil
- Pepper
- Salt

Directions:

Heat olive oil in a large saucepan over medium heat.

Add squash, carrots, leeks, and fennel and sauté for 5 minutes.

Add turmeric, ginger, garlic, pepper, and salt and sauté for 2–3 minutes.

Add coconut milk and vegetable broth. Bring to a boil, cover, and simmer for 20 minutes. Remove saucepan from heat.

Puree the soup using an immersion blender until smooth and creamy.

Serve and enjoy.

Nutritional Data: 360 calories | 28.09g carbs | 28.34g fat | 4.65g protein | 504mg sodium

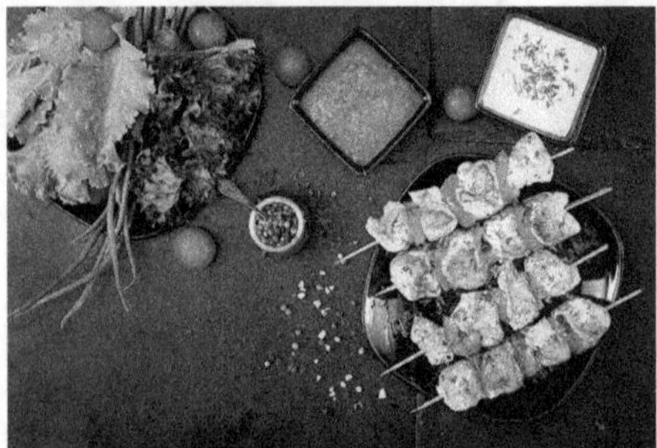

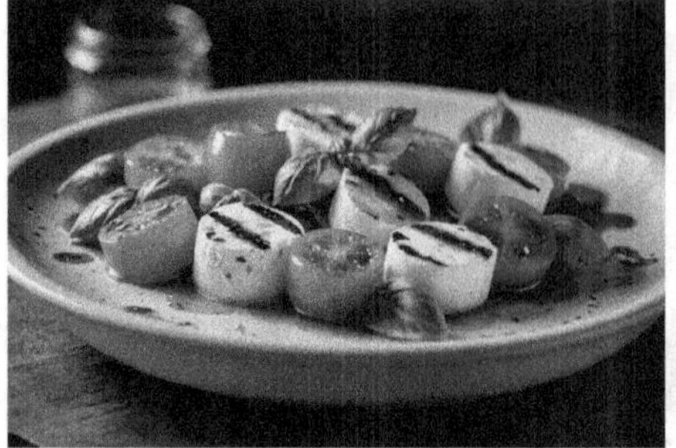

Preparation Time: 10 minutes
Cooking Time: 15 minutes
Serves: 4
Ingredients:

- 1 medium onion, cut into chunks
- 1 red bell pepper, cut into chunks
- 1 yellow bell pepper, cut into chunks
- 18 oz turkey chunks
- For marinade:
- 3 tbsp olive oil
- 1 tsp dried oregano
- ½ tsp paprika
- ½ tsp cinnamon
- 1/2 lemon, juiced
- ½ tsp pepper
- 1 tsp salt

Directions:

In a mixing bowl, add all marinade ingredients and turkey chunks and mix well.

Cover and place in refrigerator overnight.

Thread marinated turkey chunks, bell pepper, and onion onto skewers.

Place skewers onto a hot grill and cook over medium-high heat for 10–15 or until the meat is cooked through.

Serve and enjoy.

Nutritional Data: 726 calories | 5.18g carbs | 66.96g fat | 25.02g protein | 640mg sodium

Preparation Time: 10 minutes
Cooking Time: 5 minutes
Serves: 6
Ingredients:

- 20 oz cherry tomatoes, halved
- ½ tbsp honey
- 1 garlic clove, minced
- 1 lemon, juiced
- 3 tbsp balsamic vinegar
- ½ cup olive oil
- 1/3 cup basil leaves, chopped
- 10 oz mozzarella balls
- Pepper
- Salt

Directions:

In a mixing bowl, mix cherry tomatoes, basil leaves, and mozzarella balls.

In a small bowl, whisk together honey, garlic, lemon juice, vinegar, oil, pepper, and salt.

Pour dressing over salad and toss well.

Cover salad bowl and place in refrigerator for 1 hour.

Serve and enjoy.

Nutritional Data: 252 calories | 23.11g carbs | 18.34g fat | 1.65g protein | 18mg sodium

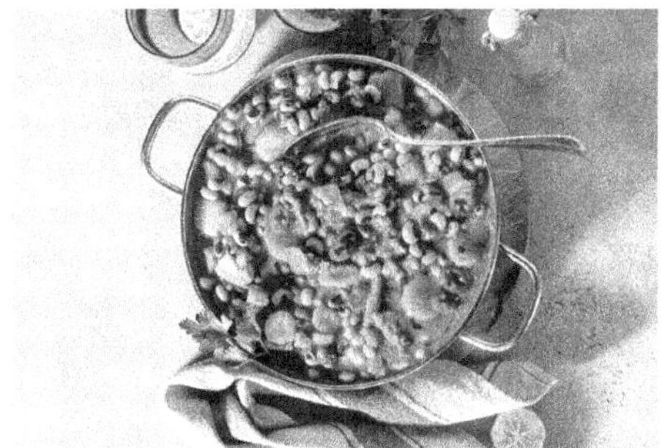

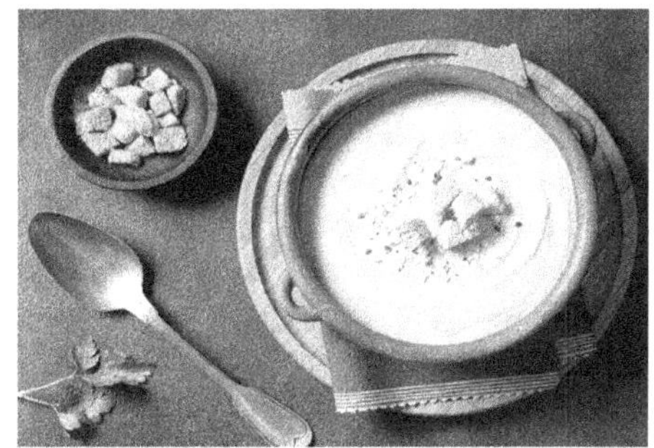

Preparation Time: 10 minutes
Cooking Time: 60 minutes
Serves: 4
Ingredients:

- 2 eggplants, cubed
- ¼ cup dates, chopped
- 14.10-oz can chickpeas, rinsed & drained
- 1 cup vegetable broth
- 14.10-oz can crushed tomatoes
- ½ tsp turmeric
- 1 tsp paprika
- 1 tsp cinnamon
- 1 tsp cumin
- 4 garlic cloves, minced
- 1 onion, diced
- 1 tbsp olive oil
- 1 tsp sea salt

Directions:

Heat olive oil in a large pot over medium heat.

Add onion and sauté for 4–5 minutes.

Add eggplant and garlic and cook for 10 minutes or until eggplant is tender.

Add turmeric, paprika, cinnamon, and cumin and stir for 2 minutes.

Add tomatoes, vegetable broth, and salt, cover, and simmer for 30 minutes.

Add chickpeas and dates, stir well, and simmer for 20 minutes.

Serve and enjoy.

Nutritional Data: 304 calories | 54.63g carbs | 7.18g fat | 11.48g protein | 1088mg sodium

Preparation Time: 10 minutes
Cooking Time: 5 minutes
Serves: 2
Ingredients:

- 1 avocado, flesh scooped out
- 1 cucumber, peeled & chopped
- 3 tbsp cilantro, chopped
- ½ lemon, juiced
- ½ cup water
- 1 jalapeno pepper, cut in half & seeds removed
- ½ tsp salt

Directions:

Add avocado, cucumber, and remaining ingredients into blender and blend until smooth and creamy.

Pour blended soup into bowl, cover, and place in refrigerator for 2 hours.

Serve chilled and enjoy.

Nutritional Data: 178 calories | 12.08g carbs | 14.96g fat | 2.74g protein | 593mg sodium

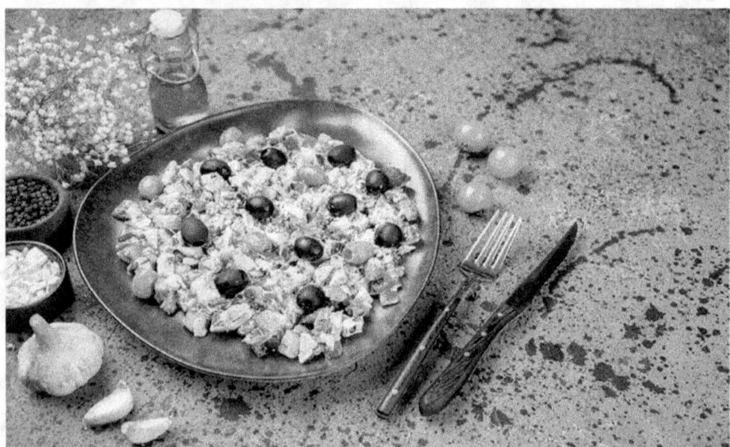

Preparation Time: 10 minutes
Cooking Time: 15 minutes
Serves: 4
Ingredients:

- For chicken:
- 1 lb chicken breast, boneless & skinless
- 1 tsp dried oregano
- 2 tsp garlic, minced
- 2 tsp dried basil
- 2 tbsp fresh parsley, chopped
- 2 tbsp red wine vinegar
- 2 tbsp water
- ¼ cup fresh lemon juice
- 2 tbsp olive oil
- Pepper
- Salt
- For salad:
- 1/3 cup olives, pitted & sliced
- 1 avocado, sliced
- 1 onion, sliced
- 2 tomatoes, diced
- 1 cucumber, diced
- 4 cups romaine lettuce leaves, chopped

Directions:

For dressing: In a small bowl, whisk together oregano, garlic, basil, parsley, vinegar, water, lemon juice, olive oil, pepper, and salt, and set aside.

In a mixing bowl, pour half the dressing, add chicken, and mix well. Cover and place in refrigerator for 30 minutes to marinate.

Spray grill pan with cooking spray and heat over medium-high heat. Add marinated chicken to the pan and cook on both sides until chicken is cooked completely.

Cut chicken into slices and place into large mixing bowl. Add olives, avocado, onion, tomatoes, cucumber, lettuce, and remaining dressing.

Mix everything well and serve.

Nutritional Data: 654 calories | 13.87g carbs | 32.64g fat | 75.27g protein | 350mg sodium

Chapter 6—Dinner Recipes

1-Grilled Salmon with Asparagus

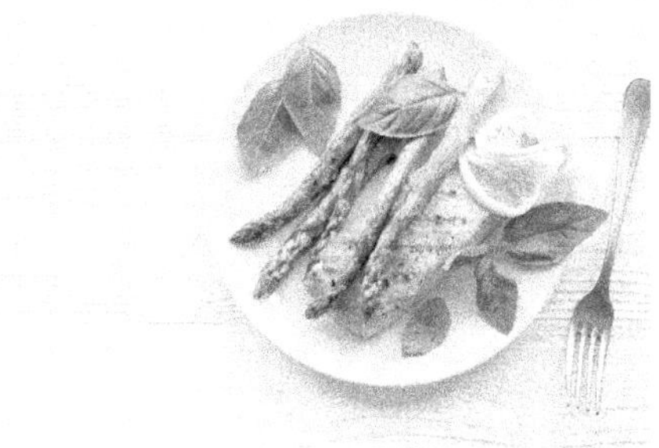

Preparation Time: 10 minutes
Cooking Time: 10 minutes
Serves: 2
Ingredients:

- 4 salmon fillets
- 1 bunch asparagus, ends trimmed
- ½ tsp garlic, minced
- 1 tbsp lemon juice
- 3 tbsp olive oil
- Pepper
- Salt

Directions:

In a mixing bowl, add salmon fillets, garlic, lemon juice, 2 tablespoons olive oil, pepper, and salt and mix to coat well. Cover the bowl and place in the refrigerator for 30 minutes to marinate salmon.

Preheat grill to medium-high heat.

Toss asparagus with remaining olive oil, pepper, and salt.

Place asparagus onto hot grill and cook for 3–4 minutes on each side. Remove from grill and set aside.

Remove salmon from marinade and place on hot grill and cook for 4–5 minutes on each side or until the salmon is cooked through.

Serve grilled salmon with asparagus.

Nutritional Data: 537 calories | 3.2g carbs | 36.46g fat | 47.11g protein | 977mg sodium

2-Vegetarian Chili

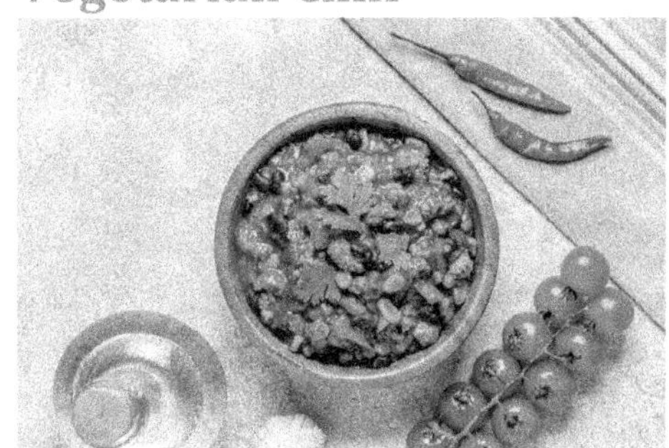

Preparation Time: 10 minutes
Cooking Time: 40 minutes
Serves: 8
Ingredients:

- 15-oz can red beans, rinsed & drained
- 15-oz can black beans, rinsed & drained
- 29-oz can tomatoes, diced
- ¼ cup cilantro, chopped
- 1 zucchini, diced
- 1 small sweet potato, peeled & diced
- 4 cups vegetable stock
- 1 ½ tsp dried oregano
- 1 ½ tsp ground cumin
- 1 tbsp chili powder
- 1 tbsp garlic, minced
- 1 small poblano pepper, diced
- 1 onion, diced
- 2 tbsp olive oil
- Pepper
- Salt

Directions:

Heat olive oil in a large pot over medium heat.

Add poblano and onion and sauté for 2–3 minutes. Add garlic, oregano, cumin, and chili powder and stir for 1 minute.

Add tomatoes, stock, red beans, black beans, pepper, and salt and stir well.

Bring to a boil, turn the heat to low, and simmer for 15–20 minutes.

Add zucchini and sweet potato and cook until tender, about 12–15 minutes.

Add cilantro and stir well. Season with pepper and salt.

Serve and enjoy.

Nutritional Data: 178 calories | 12.08g carbs | 14.96g fat | 2.74g protein | 593mg sodium

3-Lemon Herb Chicken

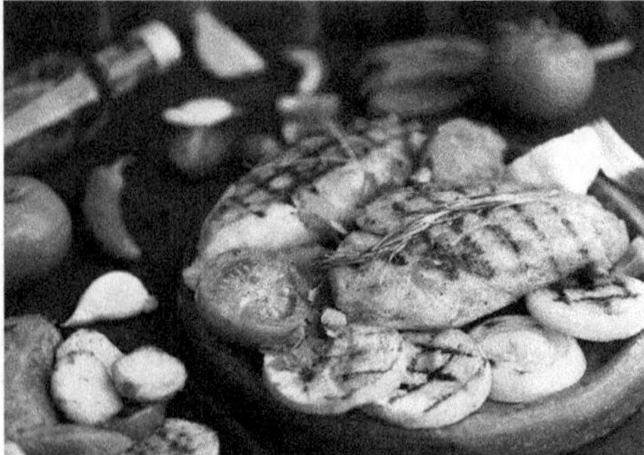

Preparation Time: 10 minutes
Cooking Time: 15 minutes
Serves: 4
Ingredients:

- 2 lbs chicken breast, trimmed
- For marinade:
- 4 tbsp lemon juice
- 4 tbsp olive oil
- ¼ tsp red pepper flakes, crushed
- ½ tsp onion powder
- ½ tsp garlic powder
- 1 tbsp dried parsley
- 1 tbsp dried basil
- ½ tsp pepper
- 1 tsp salt

Directions:

Add chicken and all marinade ingredients into large mixing bowl and mix well. Cover and place in refrigerator overnight.

Preheat grill to medium heat.

Remove chicken from marinade and place onto the hot grill and cook for 5–7 minutes on each side or until chicken is cooked through.

Serve and enjoy.

Nutritional Data: 519 calories | 2.46g carbs | 34.55g fat | 47.66g protein | 726mg sodium

4-Stuffed Bell Peppers

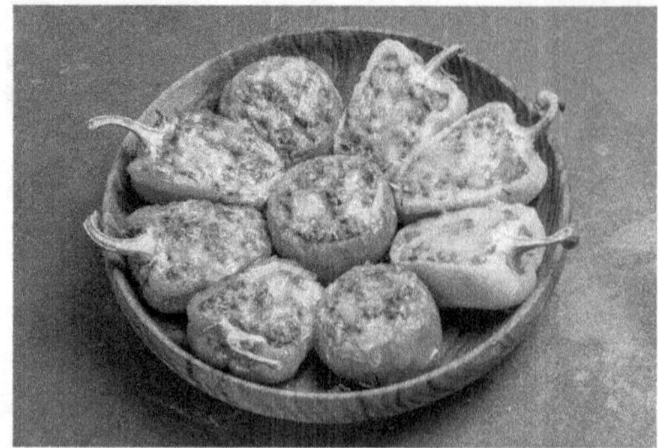

Preparation Time: 10 minutes
Cooking Time: 25 minutes
Serves: 6
Ingredients:

- 3 bell peppers, cut in half and seeds removed
- 2 tbsp harissa
- ¼ cup feta cheese, crumbled
- ½ cup cherry tomatoes, sliced
- 1/3-cup can chickpeas, rinsed
- ½ tsp oregano
- 1 tsp garlic, minced
- 1 ½ cups cooked quinoa
- ½ tsp salt

Directions:

Preheat oven to 400°F.

In a mixing bowl, mix together cooked quinoa, garlic, oregano, chickpeas, tomatoes, and salt.

Stuff the quinoa mixture in each bell pepper half.

Place stuffed bell pepper onto baking sheet and bake in preheated oven for 20–25 minutes.

Top with crumbled cheese and drizzle with harissa paste.

Serve and enjoy.

Nutritional Data: 418 calories | 26.3g carbs | 31.11g fat | 14.19g protein | 258mg sodium

5-Cauliflower-Rice Stir-Fry

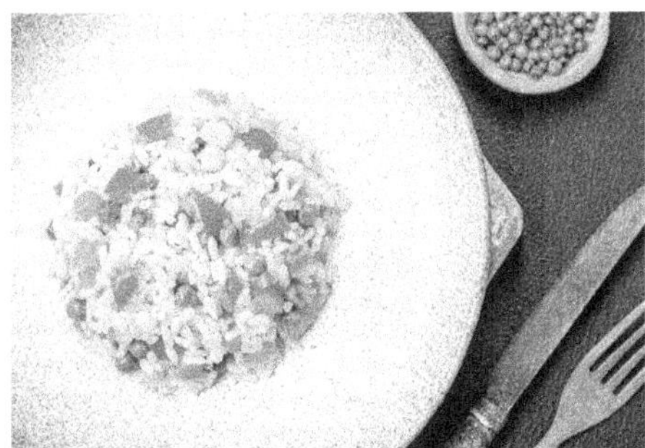

Preparation Time: 10 minutes
Cooking Time: 10 minutes
Serves: 6
Ingredients:

- 20 oz cauliflower rice
- ¼ cup green onions, chopped
- 2 tsp sesame oil
- 1 tsp chili paste
- 2 tbsp low-sodium soy sauce
- 2 cups frozen stir-fry vegetables
- 2 tsp ginger, grated
- 1 tbsp garlic, minced
- 1 tbsp olive oil
- Pepper
- Salt

Directions:

Heat olive oil in a large pan over medium heat.

Add ginger and garlic and cook for 1 minute.

Add vegetables and cauliflower rice to the pan and cook for 5–8 minutes or until vegetables are tender.

Add chili paste and soy sauce and stir well to combine. Remove pan from heat.

Drizzle with sesame oil and sprinkle with green onion. Season with pepper and salt.

Serve and enjoy.

Nutritional Data: 207 calories | 20.86g carbs | 11.04g fat | 6.65g protein | 328mg sodium

6-Baked Cod with Roasted Vegetables

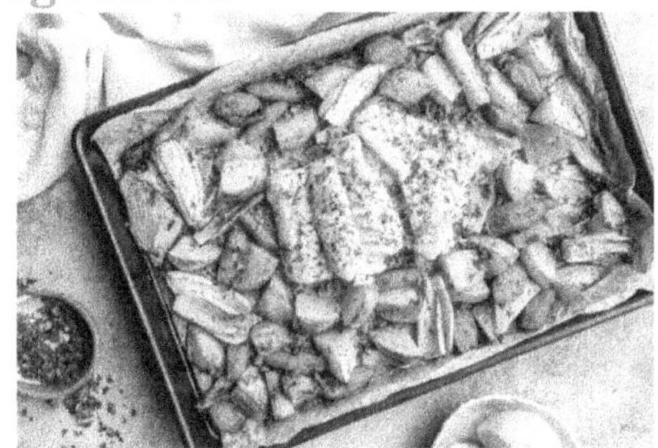

Preparation Time: 10 minutes
Cooking Time: 35 minutes
Serves: 2
Ingredients:

- 2 cod fillets
- ½ tsp dried thyme
- ½ tsp garlic powder
- 1 tbsp apple cider vinegar
- ½ lemon, juiced
- ¼ cup olive oil
- 2 cups fennel, cut into 3/4-inch pieces
- 1 cup carrots, peeled & chopped
- 2 cups potatoes, cut into 3/4-inch pieces
- Pepper
- Salt

Directions:

Preheat oven to 400°F.

Line baking sheet with parchment paper and set aside.

In a small bowl, whisk together olive oil, thyme, garlic powder, vinegar, lemon juice, pepper, and salt.

In a mixing bowl, add fennel, carrots, and potatoes. Pour half the olive oil mixture over the vegetables and toss to coat.

Spread vegetables onto baking sheet and bake in preheated oven for 20 minutes.

Remove the baking sheet from the oven then place cod fillets in the center of the baking sheet. Brush cod fillets with the remaining olive oil mixture and season with pepper and salt.

Return the baking sheet to the oven for 12–15 minutes or until the fish is opaque.

Serve and enjoy.

Nutritional Data: 502 calories | 42.29g carbs | 28.01g fat | 22.98g protein | 447mg sodium

7-Turkey Meatballs with Zoodles

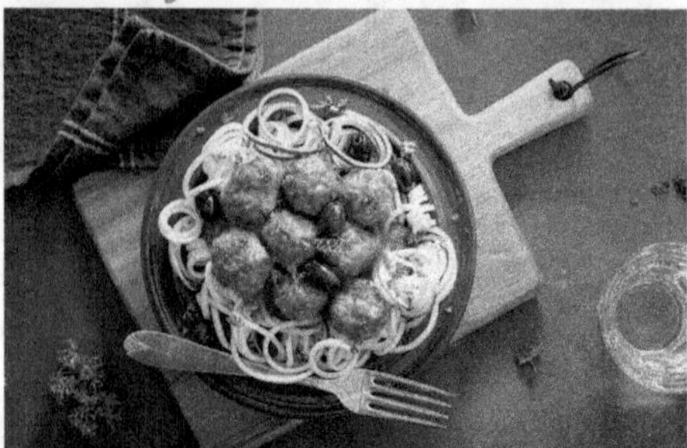

Preparation Time: 10 minutes
Cooking Time: 15 minutes
Serves: 4
Ingredients:

- 1 lb ground turkey meat
- 1 tbsp hot sauce
- ½ lemon, juiced
- 4 zucchinis, spiralized
- 3 tbsp butter
- 1 cup parsley, chopped
- ½ tsp red pepper flakes, crushed
- 1 tsp Italian seasoning
- 1 tbsp garlic, minced
- ½ cup mozzarella cheese, shredded
- Pepper
- Salt

Directions:

In a mixing bowl, mix together ground turkey meat, parsley, red pepper flakes, Italian seasoning, garlic, cheese, pepper, and salt until well combined.

Make equal shapes of balls from the meat mixture and place on a plate. Set aside.

Melt 2 tablespoons butter in a large pan over medium-low heat.

Add meatballs to the pan and cook for 8–10 minutes or until cooked through. Transfer meatballs onto a plate and set aside.

Melt remaining butter in same pan, add lemon juice, hot sauce, and zucchini noodles, and cook for 3–4 minutes. Season with pepper and salt.

Serve zucchini noodles with turkey meatballs.

Nutritional Data: 286 calories | 4.99g carbs | 17.56g fat | 28.15g protein | 397mg sodium

8-Shrimp-and-Vegetable Skewers

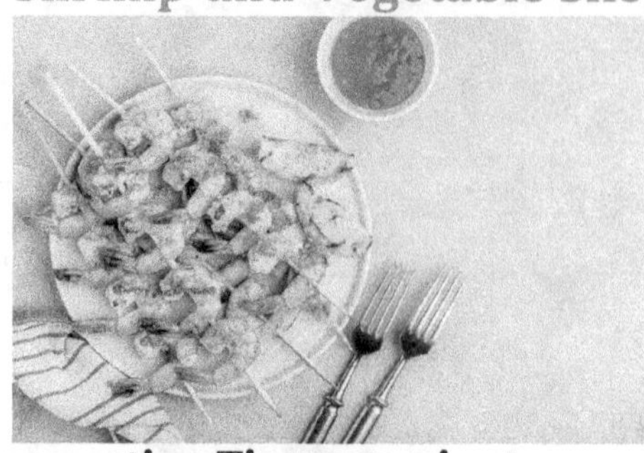

Preparation Time: 10 minutes
Cooking Time: 6 minutes
Serves: 4
Ingredients:

- 1 lb shrimp, peeled & deveined
- 1 onion, cut into 1-inch pieces
- 1 red bell pepper, cut into 1-inch pieces
- 1 yellow bell pepper, cut into 1-inch pieces
- ¼ tsp cayenne
- ½ tsp paprika
- 1 tsp dried oregano
- 2 tsp dried basil
- 1 tbsp garlic, minced
- 2 tbsp red wine vinegar
- 3 tbsp olive oil
- 1/3 cup tomato sauce
- ¾ tsp salt

Directions:

In a mixing bowl, mix together tomato sauce, oil, vinegar, garlic, basil, oregano, paprika, cayenne, and salt. Add shrimp and mix until well coated.

Cover bowl and place in refrigerator for 30 minutes to marinate the shrimp.

Preheat grill to medium heat.

Thread marinated shrimp, onion, and bell pepper onto skewers.

Place shrimp skewers onto the hot grill and cook for 3 minutes on each side.

Serve and enjoy.

Nutritional Data: 271 calories | 14.56g carbs | 12.08g fat | 25.03g protein | 1728mg sodium

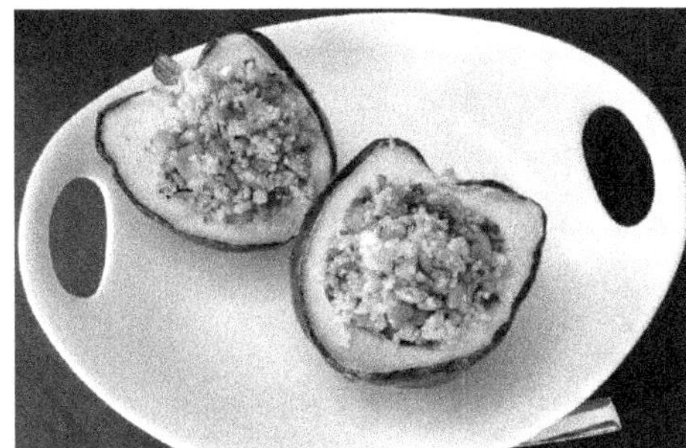

Preparation Time: 10 minutes
Cooking Time: 63 minutes
Serves: 4
Ingredients:

- 2 acorn squash, cut in half & seeds scooped out
- ½ cup gouda cheese, shredded
- 2 tsp lemon juice
- 1 tbsp maple syrup
- 2 cups cooked quinoa
- ½ onion, diced
- 1 pear, peeled & diced
- 2 celery stalks, diced
- 2 tsp olive oil

Directions:

Preheat oven to 400°F.

Brush squash with 1 teaspoon of olive oil and season with pepper and salt.

Place squash onto baking sheet and bake in preheated oven for 30–40 minutes.

Heat the remaining oil in a pan over medium heat.

Add celery, onion, and pear, and cook for 10 minutes or until onions are softened.

Add quinoa, lemon juice, and maple syrup and stir for 2–3 minutes.

Stuff the quinoa mixture into baked squash halves.

Top with cheese and bake for 10 minutes.

Serve and enjoy.

Nutritional Data: 297 calories | 50.76g carbs | 7.98g fat | 9.47g protein | 129mg sodium

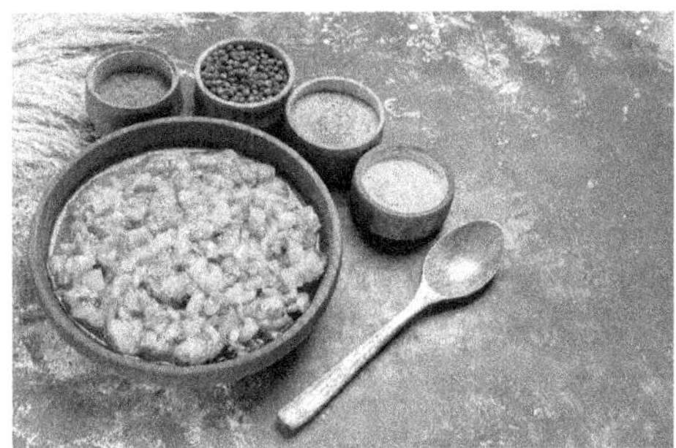

Preparation Time: 10 minutes
Cooking Time: 25 minutes
Serves: 4
Ingredients:

- 1 cup dry red lentils, rinsed
- 1 cup sweet potatoes, diced
- 2 cups spinach
- ½ tsp ginger powder
- 1 tsp garam masala
- 1 tsp curry powder
- ½ lemon, juiced
- 2 ½ cups vegetable broth
- 14.5-oz can tomatoes, diced
- 14.5-oz can coconut milk
- 1 tbsp garlic, minced
- ½ onion, diced
- 2 tbsp olive oil
- 1 tsp salt

Directions:

Heat oil in a large pot over medium heat.

Add sweet potatoes and cook for 3–4 minutes.

Add onion and sauté for 2 minutes.

Add lentils and garlic and stir for 1 minute.

Add coconut milk, ginger powder, garam masala, curry powder, lemon juice, broth, tomatoes, and salt, and stir well.

Cover and bring to a boil.

Turn heat to low and simmer for 12–15 minutes or until lentils are soft.

Add spinach and stir to combine.

Serve and enjoy

Nutritional Data: 511 calories | 45.47g carbs | 32.76g fat | 15.67g protein | 1076mg sodium

11-Spinach-and-Feta-Stuffed Chicken

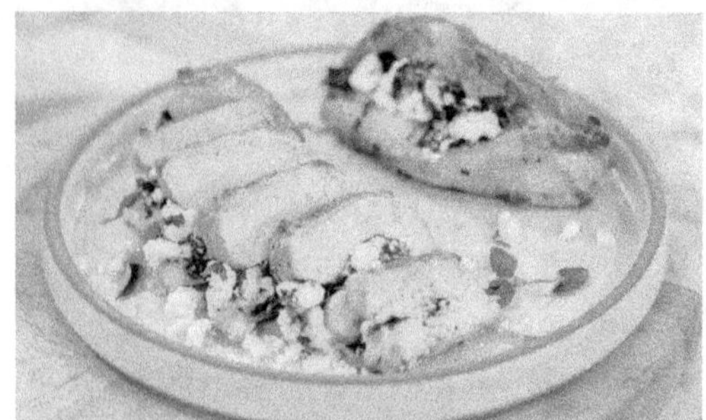

Preparation Time: 10 minutes
Cooking Time: 30 minutes
Serves: 4
Ingredients:

- 4 chicken breasts, boneless, skinless & a pocket cut into each chicken breast
- 1 tsp dried oregano
- 1 tsp garlic, minced
- ½ cup feta cheese, crumbled
- 1 cup fresh spinach, chopped
- Pepper
- Salt

Directions:

Preheat oven to 375°F.

In a mixing bowl, mix together spinach, oregano, garlic, feta, pepper, and salt.

Stuff each chicken breast with spinach mixture and secure with toothpicks.

Place stuffed chicken breasts into baking dish and bake in preheated oven for 25–30 minutes or until the chicken is cooked through.

Serve and enjoy

Nutritional Data: 556 calories | 2.51g carbs | 30.88g fat | 63.64g protein | 362mg sodium

12-Zucchini Noodles with Pesto and Cherry Tomatoes

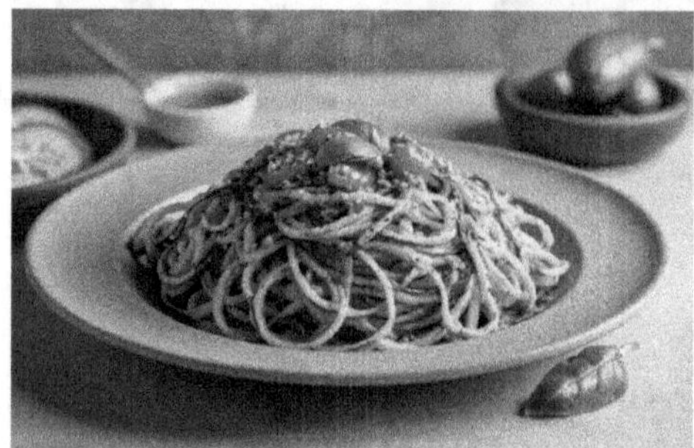

Preparation Time: 10 minutes
Cooking Time: 10 minutes
Serves: 4
Ingredients:

- 2 zucchinis, spiralized
- 1 cup cherry tomatoes
- Salt
- For pesto:
- 1/3 cup walnuts, toasted
- 4 tbsp olive oil
- 1 tbsp lemon juice
- 2 cups fresh basil leaves
- 1 garlic head, roasted & squeezed

Directions:

Add zucchini noodles and salt into colander and set aside for 20 minutes to remove excess liquid.

Add walnuts, olive oil, lemon juice, basil, and garlic into blender and blend until smooth.

Drain zucchini noodles and transfer them into large mixing bowl. Add cherry tomatoes and pesto and toss until well combined.

Serve and enjoy.

Nutritional Data: 166 calories | 1.67g carbs | 17.84g fat | 1.2g protein | 1mg sodium

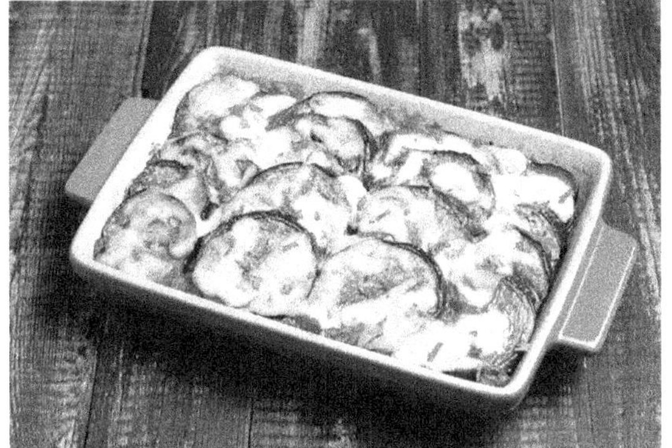

Preparation Time: 10 minutes
Cooking Time: 25 minutes
Serves: 4
Ingredients:

- 2 medium eggplants, cut into round slices
- ¼ cup basil
- ¼ cup almond flour
- ¼ cup parmesan cheese, grated
- 1 cup mozzarella cheese, grated
- 16 oz marinara sauce
- 2 tsp Italian seasoning
- 1 tbsp olive oil
- Pepper
- Salt

Directions:

Preheat oven to 400°F.

Sprinkle the eggplant slices with salt and let sit for 15 minutes. Remove excess moisture from eggplant slices using a paper towel.

Place eggplant slices onto parchment-lined baking sheet. Brush with oil and season with Italian seasoning, pepper, and salt.

Bake eggplant slices in preheated oven for 20–25 minutes or until softened.

Spray 8x8-inch baking dish with cooking spray.

Add 1/3 of the marinara sauce to the baking dish. Arrange half the eggplant slices on top of the sauce. Sprinkle half of

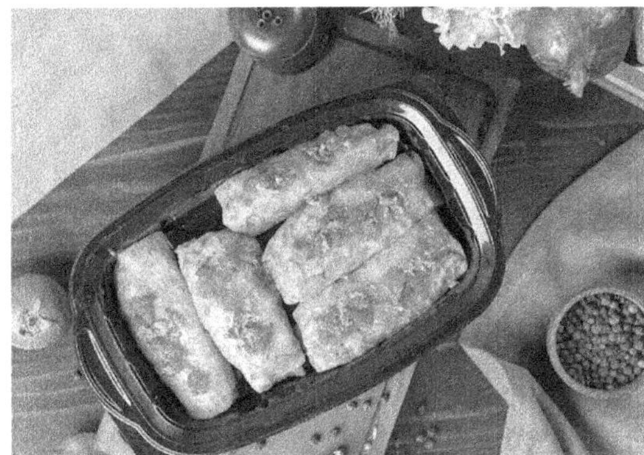

Preparation Time: 10 minutes
Cooking Time: 15 minutes
Serves: 5
Ingredients:

- 5 cabbage leaves
- 1 tsp red chili sauce
- 1 tsp low-sodium soy sauce
- 1/3 cup tofu, grated
- 1 Thai chili, chopped
- ¼ cup broccoli, chopped
- 1/3 cup carrot, grated
- 1/3 cup cabbage, grated
- 1 tbsp ginger, chopped
- 1 tbsp garlic, chopped
- ½ onion, chopped
- 2 tbsp olive oil
- Pepper
- Salt

Directions:

Add cabbage leaves into boiling water and cook until tender. Remove the leaves and place them on a paper towel.

Heat 1 tablespoon of oil in a pan over medium heat.

Add garlic and ginger and sauté for 30 seconds.

Add onion and sauté until onion is softened.

Add grated cabbage, carrot, broccoli, Thai chili, tofu, soy sauce, red chili sauce, pepper, and salt, and cook for 3–5 minutes. Remove pan from heat.

Place a cabbage leaf on a board and add 1 tablespoon of stuffing in the middle of the mozzarella cheese on top of the eggplant slices.

Add the remaining sauce and eggplant slices, and then sprinkle the remaining mozzarella cheese on top.

Mix together the parmesan cheese and almond flour and sprinkle on top.

Cover the baking dish with foil and bake at 400°F for 20 minutes.

Garnish with basil and serve.

Nutritional Data: 230 calories | 28.46g carbs | 7.36g fat | 15.37g protein | 907mg sodium

the cabbage leaf. Fold the sides to the middle then roll the leaf until the stuffing is enclosed inside.

Heat the remaining oil in a pan over medium heat.

Sear cabbage rolls on both sides and serve with sauce.

Nutritional Data: 102 calories | 10.59g carbs | 6.6g fat | 2.2g protein | 152mg sodium

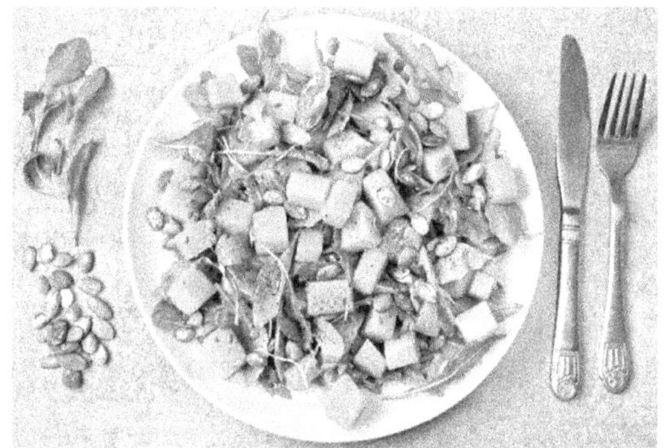

Preparation Time: 10 minutes
Cooking Time: 20 minutes
Serves: 6
Ingredients:

- 1 large butternut squash, peeled & cut into 1-inch cubes
- 1/3 cup pumpkin seeds, roasted
- ¼ cup dried cranberries
- 4 cups kale, chopped
- 1 onion, sliced
- 1/8 tsp pepper
- ¼ tsp salt
- For dressing:
- 1/3 cup olive oil
- 1 tbsp honey
- 2 tbsp apple cider vinegar
- ½ pear, chopped
- ½ avocado, chopped
- Salt

Directions:

Preheat oven to 400°F.

In a bowl, toss squash with oil, pepper, and salt.

Spread squash onto the parchment-lined baking sheet and roast in preheated oven for 15–20 minutes or until lightly golden brown from all sides.

Add all dressing ingredients into blender and blend until smooth.

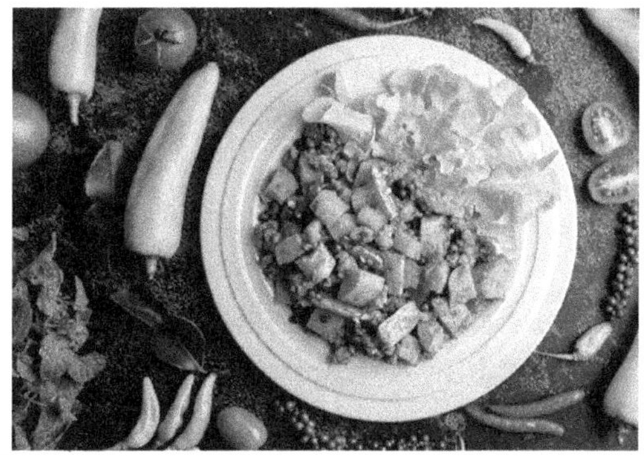

Preparation Time: 10 minutes
Cooking Time: 15 minutes
Serves: 4
Ingredients:

- 14 oz extra-firm tofu, pressed, drained & cut into 1-inch cubes
- 1 cup baby carrots, cut lengthwise
- 2 ½ cups green beans, cut into 1-inch pieces
- 3 tbsp olive oil
- 1 tbsp cornstarch
- ½ tsp kosher salt
- For sauce:
- 1 ½ tbsp ginger, grated
- 1 tbsp sesame oil
- 2 tbsp water
- 1 tbsp cornstarch
- 3 tbsp coconut sugar
- ¼ tsp red pepper flakes, crushed
- 3 tbsp low-sodium soy sauce
- 1 tbsp rice vinegar
- 1 ½ tbsp garlic, minced
- 1 ½ tbsp ginger, grated

Directions:

In a bowl, toss tofu cubes with cornstarch and salt until well coated.

Add all sauce ingredients into blender and blend until smooth. Set aside.

Heat 2 tablespoons of oil in a pan over medium-high heat.

Add tofu and fry for 4–7 minutes or until brown on all sides. Add 2 tablespoons of prepared sauce and cook for 2–3 minutes

In a large mixing bowl, add kale and dressing and rub dressing to the kale. Add roasted squash, pumpkin seeds, cranberries, and onion, and mix well.

Season salad with pepper and salt.

Serve and enjoy.

Nutritional Data: 207 calories | 11.33g carbs | 17.76g fat | 3.48g protein | 121mg sodium

more. Transfer tofu to a plate.

Add the remaining 1 tablespoon of oil to the pan. Add green beans and carrots and cook for 3–4 minutes.

Return tofu to the pan along with the remaining sauce and cook for 1–2 minutes more.

Serve and enjoy.

Nutritional Data: 315 calories | 21.09g carbs | 21.97g fat | 12.1g protein | 485mg sodium

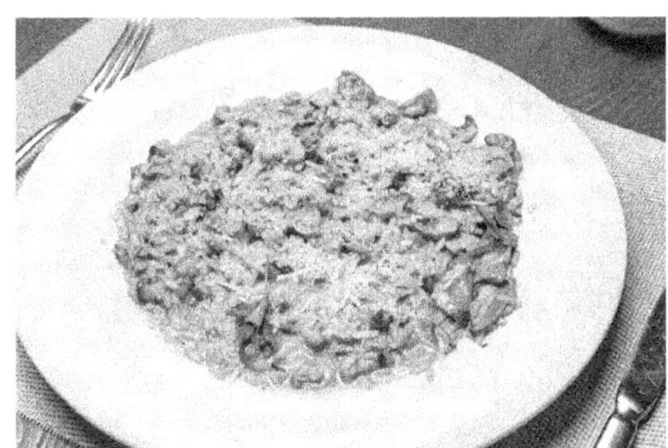

Preparation Time: 10 minutes
Cooking Time: 30 minutes
Serves: 2
Ingredients:

- ¾ cup Arborio rice
- 2 cups spinach
- 4 tbsp parsley, chopped
- ½ lemon, juiced
- 2 cups vegetable stock
- ¼ cup dried mushrooms, soaked in water for 30 minutes
- 2 garlic cloves, minced
- 4 shallots, peeled & diced
- 1 celery rib, diced
- 2 tbsp olive oil
- Pepper
- Salt

Directions:

Heat oil in a large pot over medium heat.

Add garlic, celery, and shallots, and cook for 3 minutes.

Add Arborio rice, pepper, and salt, and cook for 1 minute.

Add stock and mushrooms, stir well and cook for 20–25 minutes or until stock is absorbed completely. Remove pot from heat.

Add spinach, parsley, and lemon juice and stir everything well.

Serve and enjoy.

Nutritional Data: 524 calories | 76.69g carbs | 25.3g fat | 17.44g protein | 640mg sodium

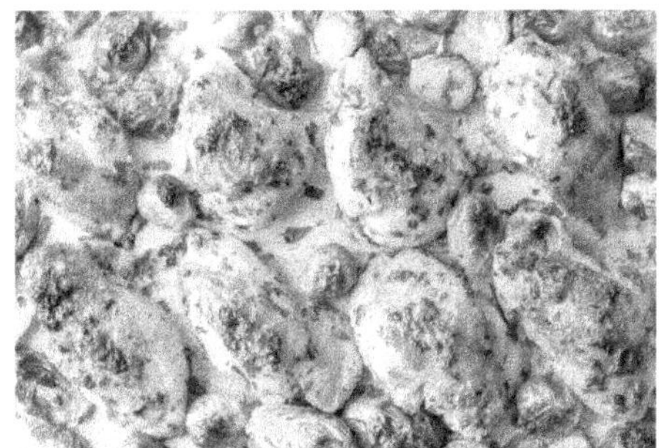

Preparation Time: 10 minutes
Cooking Time: 30 minutes
Serves: 6
Ingredients:

- 8 chicken thighs, boneless
- 2 tsp olive oil
- 1 ½ lbs Brussels sprouts, trimmed & halved
- 1/8 tsp pepper
- ½ tsp sea salt
- For marinade:
- 2 tbsp olive oil
- 1 tbsp Dijon mustard
- 2 tbsp lemon juice
- 2 tbsp parsley, chopped
- 1 tsp garlic, minced
- ½ tbsp salt

Directions:

Add chicken and all marinade ingredients into large mixing bowl and mix well. Cover bowl and place in refrigerator overnight to marinate the chicken.

In a bowl, toss Brussels sprouts with oil, pepper, and salt.

Spread Brussels sprouts and marinated chicken onto parchment-lined baking sheet and bake at 400°F for 25–30 minutes.

Serve and enjoy.

Nutritional Data: 675 calories | 11.62g carbs | 49.2g fat | 46.55g protein | 1042mg sodium

19-Cauliflower Steak with Chimichurri Sauce

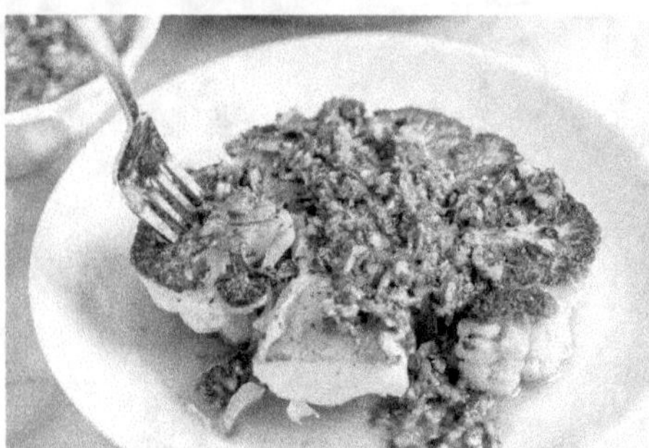

Preparation Time: 10 minutes
Cooking Time: 30 minutes
Serves: 2
Ingredients:

- 1 cauliflower head, sliced into 1-inch-thick steaks
- ½ tsp red pepper flakes, crushed
- 4 tbsp olive oil
- 2 tbsp red wine vinegar
- 1 tbsp garlic, minced
- 1 cup parsley, chopped
- 1 tsp garlic powder
- 1 tsp paprika
- 2 tbsp vegetable oil
- Pepper
- Salt

Directions:

Preheat oven to 400°F.

In a small bowl, mix together vegetable oil, garlic powder, paprika, pepper, and salt.

Brush cauliflower steaks with oil mixture and place onto baking sheet.

Roast cauliflower steaks in preheated oven for 25–30 minutes. Turn halfway through.

For sauce: In a small bowl, mix together parsley, red pepper flakes, olive oil, vinegar, garlic, pepper, and salt.

Add chimichurri sauce on top of roasted cauliflower steaks.

Serve and enjoy

Nutritional Data: 431 calories | 14.87g carbs | 41.46g fat | 4.81g protein | 63mg sodium

20-Vegetable-and-Bean Soup

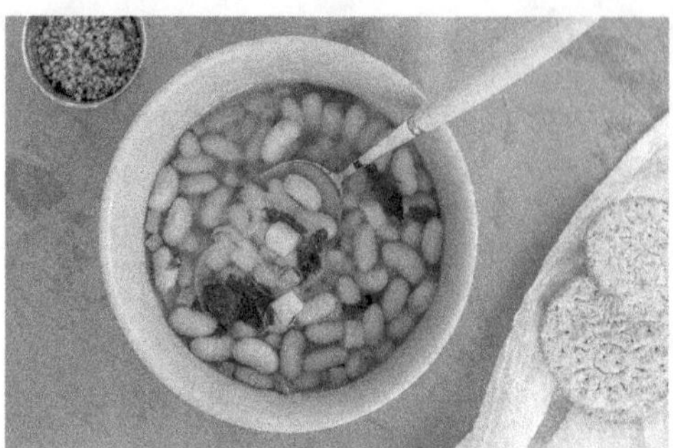

Preparation Time: 10 minutes
Cooking Time: 8 hours
Serves: 6
Ingredients:

- 1 lb dried great northern beans, soaked overnight, drained & rinsed
- 2 cups water
- 4 cups vegetable broth
- ½ tsp dried sage
- 1 tbsp garlic, minced
- 1 onion, diced
- 2 celery stalks, diced
- 3 carrots, diced
- Pepper
- Salt

Directions:

Add beans and remaining ingredients into slow cooker and stir well.

Cover and cook on high for 6–8 hours.

Season soup with pepper and salt.

Serve and enjoy.

Nutritional Data: 375 calories | 23.97g carbs | 0.47g fat | 7.07g protein | 397mg sodium

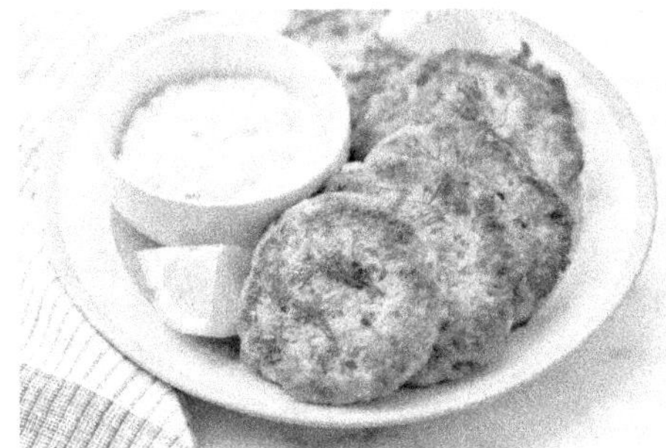

Preparation Time: 5 minutes
Cooking Time: 6 minutes
Serves: 2
Ingredients:

- 1 egg, lightly beaten
- 12 oz can salmon, drained
- 1 tbsp olive oil
- ¼ cup almond flour
- 2 tbsp green onion, chopped
- ½ tsp old bay seasoning
- ½ tsp Worcestershire sauce
- ¾ tsp Dijon mustard
- 1 ½ tbsp vegan mayonnaise
- Salt

Directions:

Add salmon into mixing bowl and break with a fork. Add remaining ingredients except olive oil and mix until well combined.

Make equal shapes of patties from the salmon mixture and place onto a plate. Place patties in refrigerator for 1 hour.

Heat olive oil in a pan over medium-high heat.

Place prepared patties into hot pan and cook for 3–4 minutes per side or until lightly golden brown.

Serve and enjoy.

Nutritional Data: 426 calories | 1.73g carbs | 27.52g fat | 40.42g protein | 911mg sodium

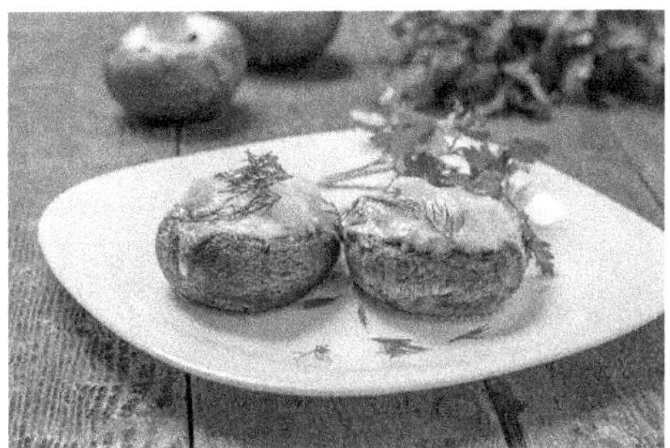

Preparation Time: 10 minutes
Cooking Time: 20 minutes
Serves: 8
Ingredients:

- 4 portobello mushrooms, stems & gills removed
- 3 oz mozzarella cheese, shredded
- 1 tsp garlic, chopped
- ½ cup parmesan cheese, grated
- 2 tbsp sour cream
- 4 oz cream cheese
- 1 can artichoke hearts, drained & chopped
- 10 oz spinach, chopped, cooked & drained
- 2 tbsp olive oil
- Pepper
- Salt

Directions:

Brush mushrooms with oil and place on a baking pan and broil on high for 5 minutes on each side.

Squeeze out excess water from cooked spinach.

In a mixing bowl, mix together spinach, garlic, parmesan cheese, sour cream, cream cheese, artichoke, pepper, and salt until well combined.

Stuff each mushroom cap with spinach mixture and top with mozzarella cheese.

Bake stuff mushrooms at 375°F for 12–15 minutes.

Serve and enjoy

Nutritional Data: 138 calories | 6.11g carbs | 9.69g fat | 8.17g protein | 291mg sodium

23-Pumpkin-and-Lentil Soup

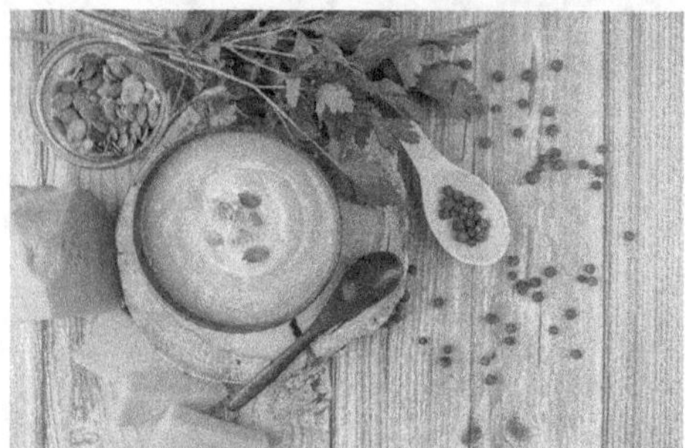

Preparation Time: 10 minutes
Cooking Time: 8 hours 5 minutes
Serves: 6
Ingredients:

- 1 cup dried red split lentils
- 2 cups vegetable stock
- 1 can coconut milk
- 2 tbsp tomato puree
- 1 tbsp olive oil
- 2 tbsp curry paste
- 1 tsp ginger, grated
- 1 tsp garlic, minced
- 1 small pumpkin, peeled & cut into small cubes
- 1 onion, chopped
- Pepper
- Salt

Directions:

Heat olive oil in a pan over medium heat.

Add pumpkin and onion and cook for 3–4 minutes. Add tomato puree, curry paste, ginger, and garlic, and cook for 1 minute more.

Transfer the pumpkin mixture into slow cooker. Add lentils, stock, and coconut milk and stir well.

Cover slow cooker with a lid and cook on low for 8 hours.

Puree the soup using an immersion blender until smooth and creamy. Season with pepper and salt.

Serve and enjoy.

Nutritional Data: 507 calories | 37.45g carbs | 33.35g fat | 22.47g protein | 301mg sodium

24-Coconut-Curry Chicken Skewers

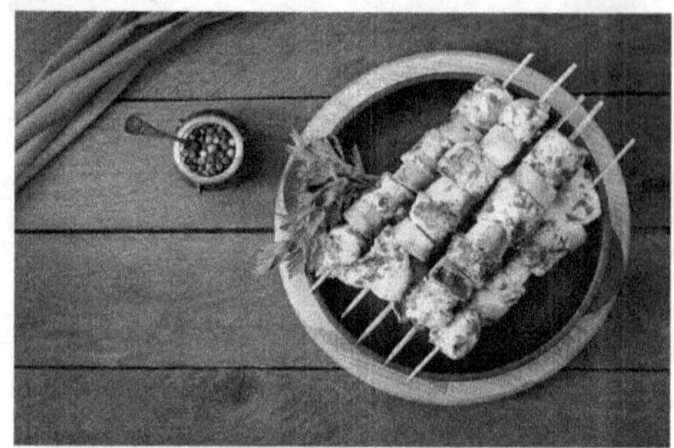

Preparation Time: 10 minutes
Cooking Time: 10 minutes
Serves: 8
Ingredients:

- 1 ½ lbs chicken breast, cut into 1-inch pieces
- 1 tsp garlic powder
- 1 tsp ginger paste
- 1 tsp curry powder
- 2 tbsp curry paste
- 2 tbsp lime juice
- 1 cup coconut milk
- Pepper
- Salt

Directions:

In a mixing bowl, add chicken pieces and remaining ingredients and mix everything well. Cover and place in refrigerator for 1 hour to marinate.

Thread marinated chicken pieces onto skewers.

Spray grill pan with cooking spray and heat over medium heat.

Place chicken skewers onto the hot grill pan and cook for 3–5 minutes on each side or until the chicken is cooked through.

Serve and enjoy

Nutritional Data: 138 calories | 6.11g carbs | 9.69g fat | 8.17g protein | 291mg sodium

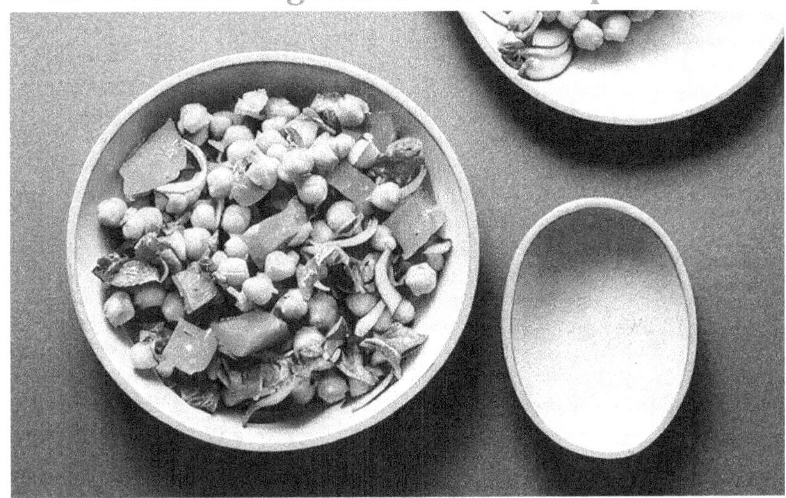

Preparation Time: 10 minutes
Cooking Time: 25 minutes
Serves: 4
Ingredients:

- ½ onion, cut into chunks
- 2 carrots, peeled & cut into ½-inch chunks
- 2 cups cauliflower florets
- 12 oz sweet potato, peeled & cut into ½-inch chunks
- 4 cups spinach
- 14-oz can chickpeas, drained & rinsed
- ½ tsp pepper
- ½ tsp garlic powder
- ¾ tsp ground cumin
- ¾ tsp paprika
- 1 ½ tsp curry powder
- 2 tbsp olive oil
- 1 tsp kosher salt

Directions:

Preheat oven to 425°F.

Lightly spray baking sheet with cooking spray and set aside.

In a large mixing bowl, toss sweet potatoes, carrots, cauliflower, and onion with 1 tablespoon of olive oil.

In a small bowl, mix together curry powder, pepper, garlic powder, cumin, paprika, and kosher salt.

Sprinkle ¾ of the curry powder mixture over vegetables and toss to coat.

In a separate bowl, toss chickpeas with the remaining curry powder mixture and olive oil.

Spread vegetables onto baking sheet and roast in preheated oven for 15 minutes.

Add chickpeas to vegetables and mix well. Roast vegetable-chickpea mixture for 10 minutes more.

Divide spinach between four serving bowls and top each with the mixture of roasted vegetables and chickpeas.

Serve and enjoy.

Nutritional Data: 279 calories | 39.8g carbs | 10.25g fat | 11.84g protein | 860mg sodium

1-Mixed Berry Parfait

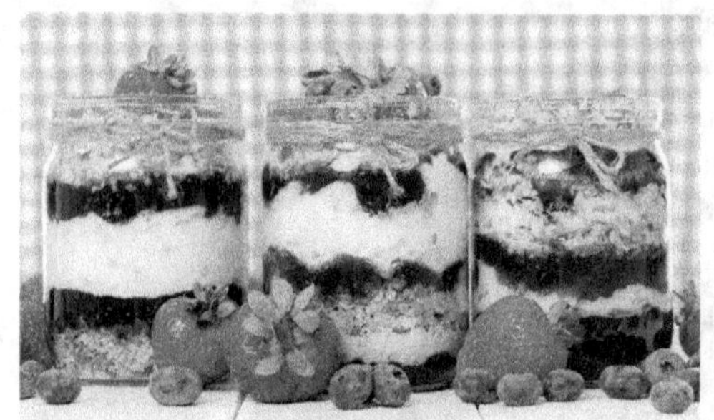

Preparation Time: 5 minutes
Cooking Time: 5 minutes
Serves: 3
Ingredients:

- 1 ½ cups Greek yogurt
- 2 cups mixed berries
- 1 ½ cups granola
- 1 tsp cinnamon
- 1 tsp vanilla

Directions:

In a mixing bowl, mix together yogurt, cinnamon, and vanilla.

Add ¼ cup yogurt to the bottom of three serving jars.

Top with ¼ berries, and granola, and repeat.

Cover and place in refrigerator until ready to serve.

Nutritional Data: 827 calories | 110.01g carbs | 33.75g fat | 21.93g protein | 481mg sodium

2-Chia Seed Pudding

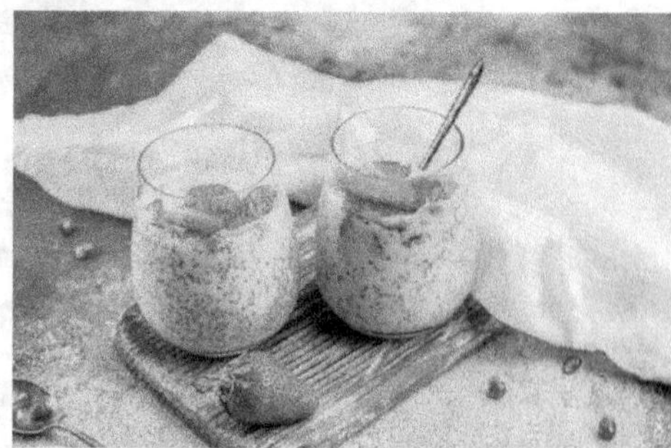

Preparation Time: 5 minutes
Cooking Time: 5 minutes
Serves: 2
Ingredients:

- 14.5-oz can full-fat coconut milk
- 6 tbsp chia seeds
- 1 tbsp honey
- ¼ tsp ginger powder
- ¼ tsp cardamom powder
- ¼ tsp cinnamon powder
- 1 ½ tsp turmeric powder
- Pinch of pepper

Directions:

Add coconut milk, honey, ginger powder, cardamom powder, cinnamon powder, turmeric powder, and pepper into blender and blend until smooth.

Pour blended mixture into glass jar. Add chia seeds and stir well. Cover the jar with a lid and place it in the refrigerator for 4 hours.

Stir well and serve

Nutritional Data: 566 calories | 27.97g carbs | 51.91g fat | 6.94g protein | 35mg sodium

3-Baked Apples

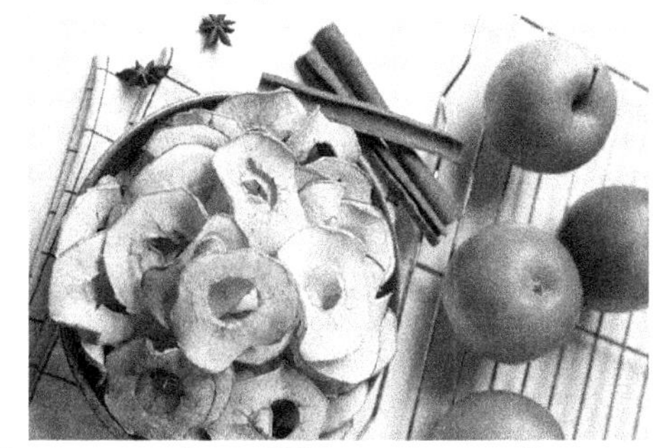

Preparation Time: 10 minutes
Cooking Time: 30 minutes
Serves: 4
Ingredients:

- 4 medium apples, sliced
- ½ tsp cinnamon
- 1 tbsp coconut oil, melted

Directions:

Preheat oven to 375°F.

In a mixing bowl, toss apple slices with cinnamon and melted coconut oil until well coated.

Add apple slices into baking dish and bake in preheated oven for 28–30 minutes or until tender.

Serve and enjoy.

Nutritional Data: 125 calories | 25.4g carbs | 3.71g fat | 0.49g protein | 2mg sodium

4-Banana Ice Cream

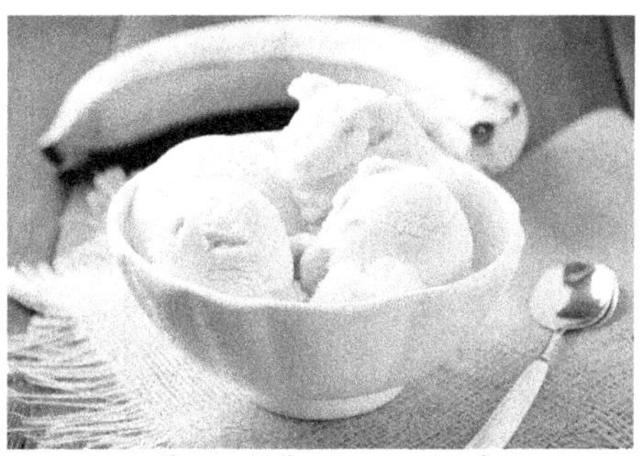

Preparation Time: 5 minutes
Cooking Time: 5 minutes
Serves: 2
Ingredients:

- 2 cups frozen banana chunks
- 1/8 tsp vanilla
- 1 tbsp unsweetened almond milk

Directions:

Add frozen banana chunks, vanilla, and almond milk into blender and blend until you get ice-cream consistency.

Serve immediately and enjoy

Nutritional Data: 350 calories | 89.02g carbs | 1.9g fat | 3.94g protein | 8mg sodium

5-Dark Chocolate Bark

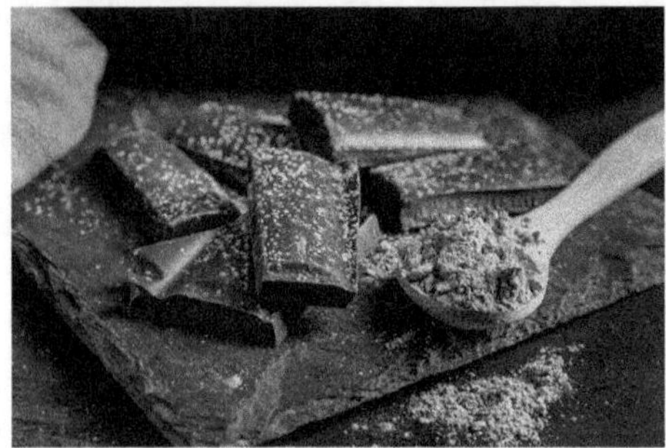

Preparation Time: 10 minutes
Cooking Time: 5 minutes
Serves: 8
Ingredients:

- 1/3 cup dark cocoa powder
- ½ tsp vanilla
- ¾ cup unsweetened shredded coconut
- ¾ cup almond butter
- ¼ cup honey
- ¼ cup coconut oil
- 1/8 tsp sea salt

Directions:

Line baking sheet with parchment paper and set aside.

Add coconut oil to a small saucepan and melt over low heat.

In a mixing bowl, mix together melted coconut oil, cocoa powder, vanilla, almond butter, honey, and sea salt until well combined.

Pour the mixture onto the parchment-lined baking sheet and spread evenly. Place in the freezer for 30 minutes or until set.

Break into pieces and serve.

Nutritional Data: 248 calories | 16.08g carbs | 20.33g fat | 5.75g protein | 117mg sodium

6-Coconut Macaroons

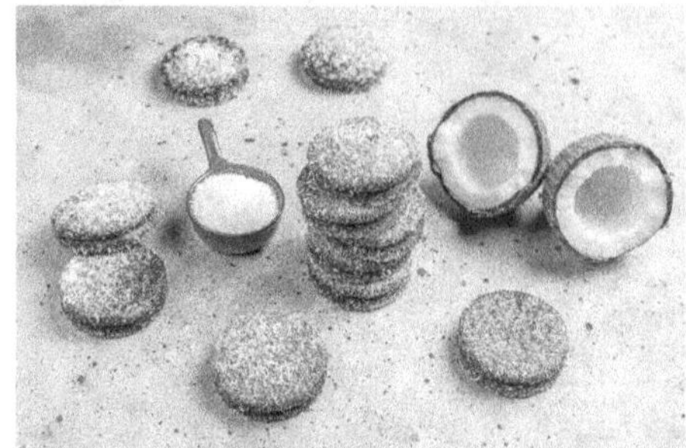

Preparation Time: 10 minutes
Cooking Time: 14 minutes
Serves: 9 macaroons
Ingredients:

- 1 ¼ cups unsweetened coconut flakes
- ¼ cup honey
- 3 tbsp coconut oil, softened
- 2 tbsp coconut flour

Directions:

Preheat oven to 350°F.

Line baking sheet with parchment paper and set aside.

Add coconut flakes, honey, coconut oil, and coconut flour into food processor and process until a thick and sticky mixture forms.

Using a cookie scoop, scoop balls of coconut mixture onto the baking sheet and bake in preheated oven for 12–14 minutes. Remove from oven and allow to cool completely.

Serve and enjoy.

Nutritional Data: 122 calories | 14.01g carbs | 7.85g fat | 0.42g protein | 38mg sodium

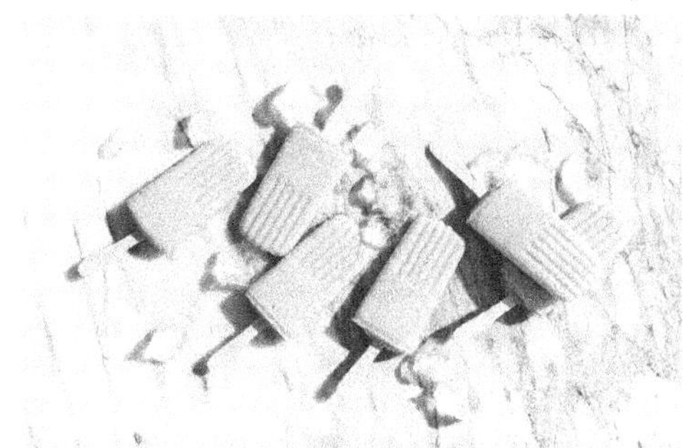

Preparation Time: 5 minutes
Cooking Time: 5 minutes
Serves: 10
Ingredients:

- 1 ½ cups full-fat coconut milk
- ¼ cup honey
- ¼ tsp pepper
- 1 ½ tsp ground ginger
- 1 ½ tsp ground turmeric
- 1 ½ cups unsweetened almond milk

Directions:

Add coconut milk, honey, pepper, ground ginger, ground turmeric, and almond milk into blender and blend until well combined.

Pour the blended mixture into popsicle mold and place it in the freezer overnight.

Serve and enjoy.

Nutritional Data: 129 calories | 12.96g carbs | 9.06g fat | 1.17g protein | 32mg sodium

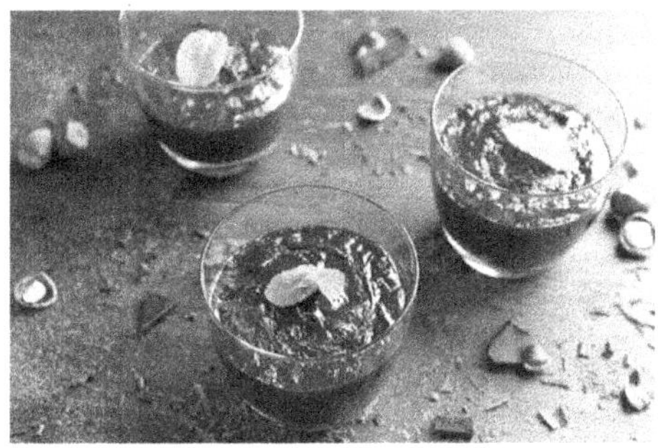

Preparation Time: 5 minutes
Cooking Time: 5 minutes
Serves: 2
Ingredients:

- 2 avocados, flesh scooped out
- 1 ½ tsp vanilla
- 6 tbsp unsweetened almond milk
- 6 tbsp maple syrup
- 6 tbsp unsweetened cocoa powder
- 1/8 tsp salt

Directions:

Add avocados, vanilla, almond milk, maple syrup, cocoa powder, and salt into blender and blend until smooth.

Pour blended mixture into air-tight container and place in the freezer for 1 hour.

Serve and enjoy.

Nutritional Data: 545 calories | 71.43g carbs | 32.19g fat | 7.26g protein | 212mg sodium

9-Almond Flour Cookies

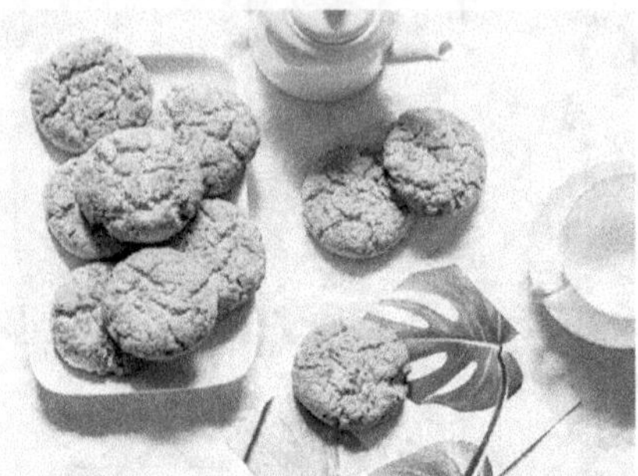

Preparation Time: 10 minutes
Cooking Time: 15 minutes
Serves: 10
Ingredients:

- 2 eggs
- 2 cups almond flour
- 1 tsp almond extract
- ¾ cup Swerve
- 4 tbsp butter, softened

Directions:

Preheat oven to 350°F.

Add butter and sweetener in a mixing bowl and beat using an immersion blender until the butter is creamy.

Add eggs and almond extract and beat until smooth.

Add almond flour and mix until well combined.

Scoop out the batter onto a parchment-lined sheet pan into 20 cookies.

Bake cookies in preheated oven for 15 minutes. Remove cookies from oven and allow to cool completely.

Serve and enjoy.

Nutritional Data: 69 calories | 0.28g carbs | 6.71g fat | 1.92g protein | 108mg sodium

10-Pineapple Coconut Sorbet

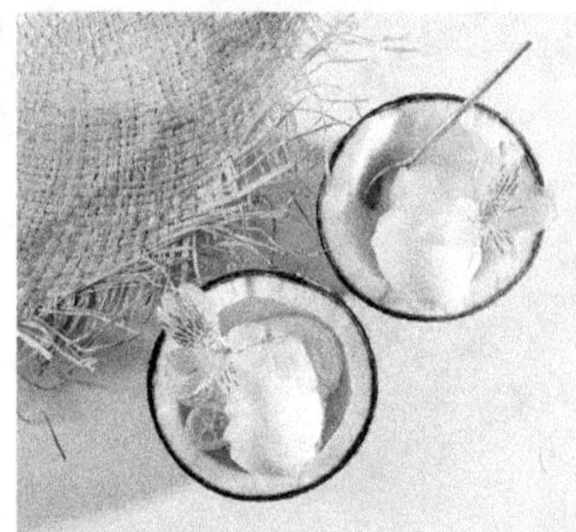

Preparation Time: 5 minutes
Cooking Time: 5 minutes
Serves: 4
Ingredients:

- 3 cups frozen pineapple chunks
- 1 tbsp honey
- 14.5 oz full-fat coconut milk

Directions:

Add pineapple, honey, and coconut milk into a blender and blend until smooth.

Pour pineapple mixture into air-tight container and place in the freezer for 3–4 hours.

Serve and enjoy.

Nutritional Data: 410 calories | 50.81g carbs | 24.69g fat | 3.1g protein | 19mg sodium

11-Berry Sorbet

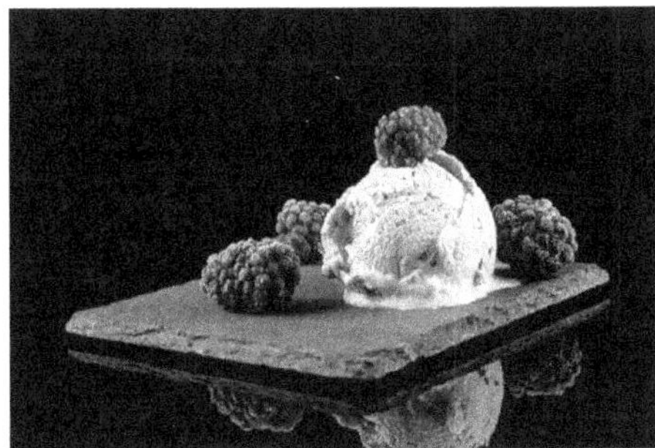

Preparation Time: 5 minutes
Cooking Time: 5 minutes
Serves: 4
Ingredients:

- 2 ½ cups mixed frozen berries
- 2 tbsp maple syrup
- 2 tsp lemon juice

Directions:

Add mixed berries, maple syrup, and lemon juice into blender and blend until smooth and creamy.

Pour blended mixture into air-tight container and place in the freezer for 2–3 hours.

Serve and enjoy.

Nutritional Data: 100 calories | 21.77g carbs | 0.18g fat | 3.27g protein | 41mg sodium

12-Pumpkin Pie Bites

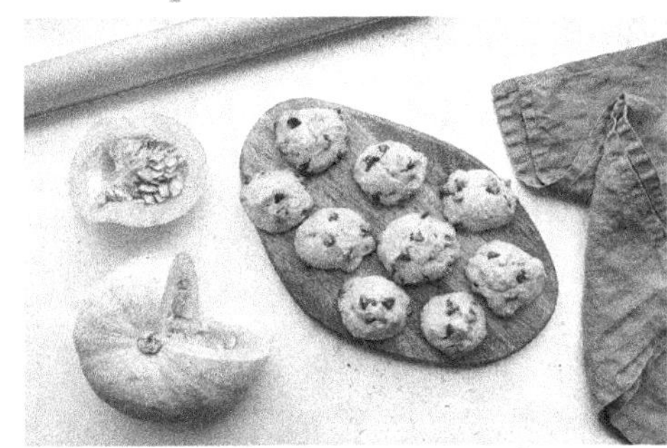

Preparation Time: 10 minutes
Cooking Time: 5 minutes
Serves: 20 Bites
Ingredients:

- ¼ cup pumpkin puree
- 2 tsp pumpkin pie spice
- ½ tsp ground cinnamon
- 1 tbsp chia seeds
- ¾ cup old-fashioned oats
- ½ cup creamy peanut butter
- ¼ cup honey

Directions:

Add oats into a blender and blend until powder forms.

Transfer the oat powder to a mixing bowl.

Add remaining ingredients and mix until well combined.

Make equal shapes of balls from the mixture and place onto a parchment-lined plate. Place in refrigerator for 15 minutes or until firm.

Serve and enjoy.

Nutritional Data: 70 calories | 7.3g carbs | 4.46g fat | 2.64g protein | 27mg sodium

13-Almond Butter Cups

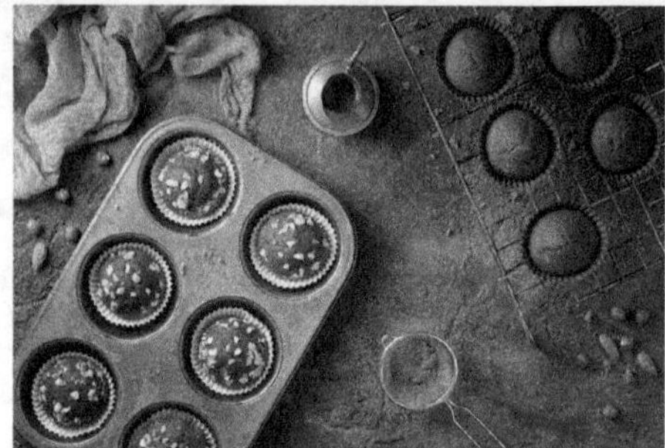

Preparation Time: 5 minutes
Cooking Time: 5 minutes
Serves: 12
Ingredients:

- ½ cup almond butter
- ½ tsp vanilla
- 1 tbsp coconut oil
- ½ cup chocolate chips
- Salt

Directions:

Add almond butter, coconut oil, and chocolate chips in a microwave-safe bowl and microwave for 60–90 seconds or until melted.

Remove bowl from microwave and add vanilla and pinch of salt. Stir well.

Pour melted mixture into mini silicone muffin molds and place in refrigerator for 6 hours.

Serve and enjoy.

Nutritional Data: 101 calories | 5.67g carbs | 8.17g fat | 2.47g protein | 46mg sodium

14-Cinnamon-Roasted Almonds

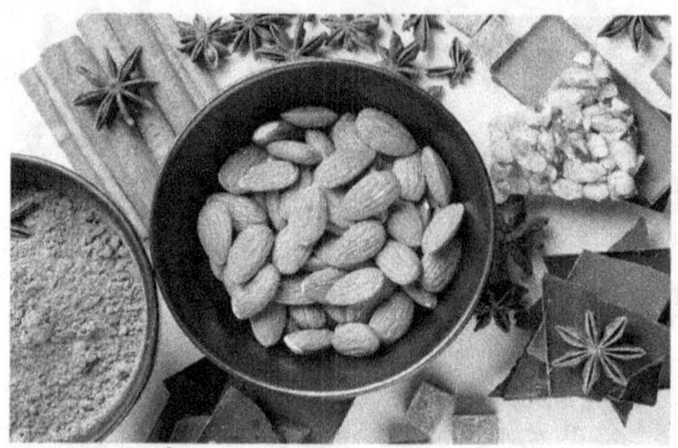

Preparation Time: 5 minutes
Cooking Time: 10 minutes
Serves: 8
Ingredients:

- 2 cups almonds
- 1 tsp ground cinnamon
- 1 tbsp honey
- 1 tbsp olive oil
- ½ tsp salt

Directions:

Preheat oven to 350°F.

Add almonds and remaining ingredients into mixing bowl and mix until almonds are coated.

Spread almonds onto a baking sheet and bake in preheated oven for 10 minutes. Remove from oven and let it cool completely.

Serve and enjoy.

Nutritional Data: 25 calories | 2.49g carbs | 1.84g fat | 0.08g protein | 146mg sodium

15-Coconut Flour Banana Bread

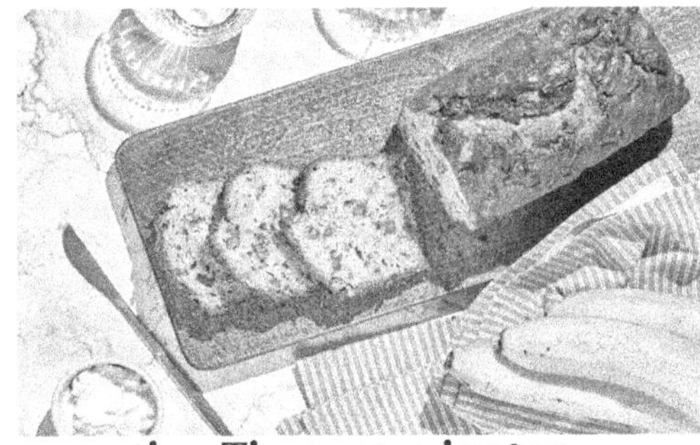

Preparation Time: 10 minutes
Cooking Time: 40 minutes
Serves: 10
Ingredients:

- 4 eggs
- ½ cup coconut flour
- 1 tsp coconut oil
- ½ tsp lemon juice
- 1 tbsp maple syrup
- 3 tbsp coconut sugar
- ½ tsp ground cinnamon
- 1 tsp vanilla
- 1 ½ tsp baking powder
- 1/3 cup tapioca flour
- 1 cup mashed bananas
- ¼ tsp sea salt

Directions:

Preheat oven to 350°F.

Line loaf pan with parchment paper and set aside.

In a medium bowl, mix coconut flour, baking powder, cinnamon, tapioca flour, and salt.

In a mixing bowl, add eggs, coconut oil, coconut sugar, maple syrup, and vanilla and beat using an immersion blender for 1–2 minutes.

Add coconut flour mixture and mashed bananas and beat until just combined.

Pour batter into the prepared loaf pan and bake in preheated oven for 40 minutes. Remove from oven and allow to cool completely.

Slice and serve.

Nutritional Data: 127 calories | 18.39g carbs | 4.52g fat | 4.08g protein | 113mg sodium

16-Lemon Poppy Seed Muffins

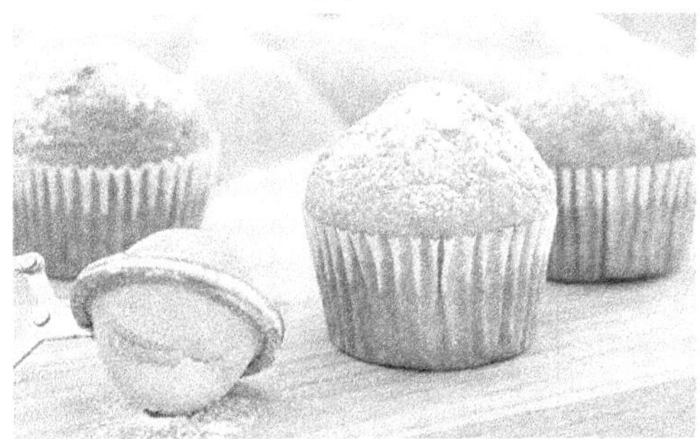

Preparation Time: 10 minutes
Cooking Time: 20 minutes
Serves: 12
Ingredients:

- 3 eggs
- 2 tbsp poppy seeds
- 3 ½ cups almond flour
- ¾ tsp baking soda
- ¾ tsp baking powder
- 1 tsp vanilla
- 2 tbsp lemon juice
- 2 lemons, zest grated
- ¾ cup Greek yogurt
- ½ cup maple syrup
- ¼ tsp salt

Directions:

Preheat oven to 350°F.

Line muffin pan with muffin liners and set aside.

In a mixing bowl, whisk eggs, baking soda, baking powder, vanilla, lemon zest, lemon juice, yogurt, maple syrup, and salt until combined.

Add poppy seeds and almond flour and mix well.

Spoon batter into the prepared muffin pan and bake for 20 minutes. Remove from oven and let it cool for 10 minutes.

Serve and enjoy.

Nutritional Data: 87 calories | 10.91g carbs | 3.28g fat | 3.9g protein | 161mg sodium

17-Ginger Turmeric Cookies

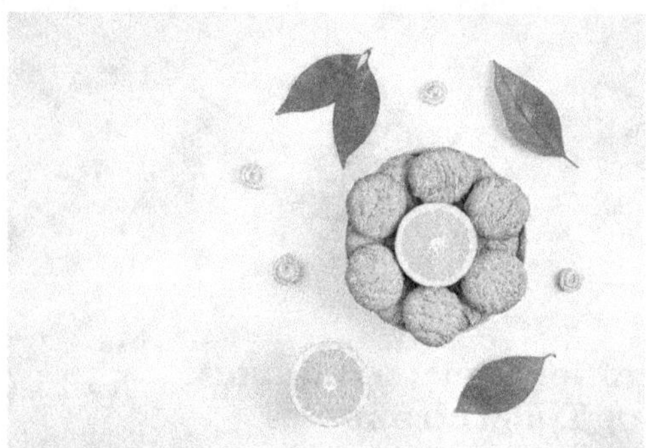

Preparation Time: 10 minutes
Cooking Time: 25 minutes
Serves: 12
Ingredients:

- 1 cup oats
- ½ cup ground almonds
- 2 tbsp almond butter
- ½ cup coconut oil, melted
- 1/3 cup maple syrup
- 1 ripe banana, mashed
- 1 tsp baking powder
- 1 ½ tsp turmeric
- 1 tsp fresh ginger, grated
- 3 tsp ground ginger
- 1 tsp cinnamon
- 1 tsp mixed spice
- 1 cup desiccated coconut
- ½ cup mixed seeds
- Sea salt

Directions:

Preheat oven to 350°F.

In a mixing bowl, mix together almond butter, melted oil, maple syrup, and mashed banana.

Add remaining ingredients and mix until well combined.

Make equal shapes of balls from the mixture and place onto a parchment-lined baking sheet.

Bake cookies in preheated oven for 20–25 minutes.

Serve and enjoy.

Nutritional Data: 190 calories | 16.32g carbs | 14.73g fat | 3.49g protein | 30mg sodium

18-Cranberry Almond Energy Bites

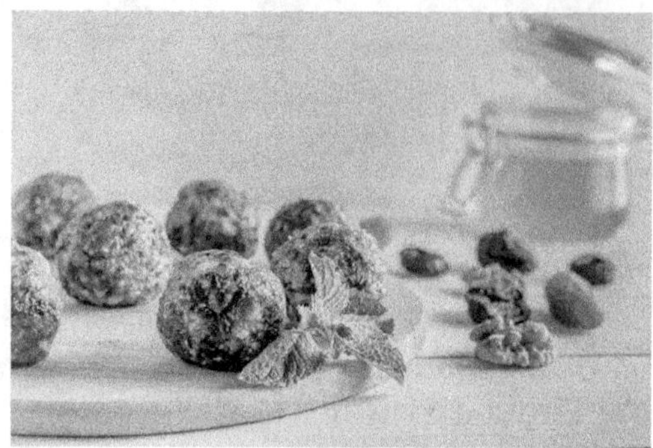

Preparation Time: 10 minutes
Cooking Time: 5 minutes
Serves: 6
Ingredients:

- 1 cup oats
- 1 tbsp chia seeds
- 1 tsp vanilla
- ½ cup honey
- ½ cup peanut butter
- ¼ cup almonds, sliced
- ½ cup dried cranberries, chopped

Directions:

In a mixing bowl, add oats and remaining ingredients and mix until well combined.

Make equal shapes of balls from the oat mixture and place onto a parchment-lined plate. Place in refrigerator for 15 minutes.

Serve and enjoy.

Nutritional Data: 202 calories | 42.1g carbs | 5.15g fat | 4.4g protein | 323mg sodium

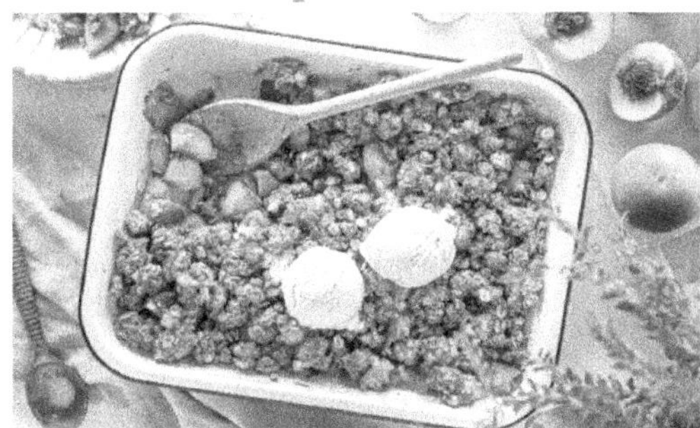

Preparation Time: 10 minutes
Cooking Time: 30 minutes
Serves: 8
Ingredients:

- 6 peaches, sliced
- 1 cup old-fashioned rolled oats
- ½ tsp cinnamon
- 1 tsp vanilla
- ¼ cup coconut oil, melted
- 1/3 cup maple syrup
- ½ cup almond flour
- ½ cup pecans, chopped
- 1 tbsp lemon juice
- 1 tbsp arrowroot powder
- ¼ tsp sea salt

Directions:

Preheat oven to 375°F.

Lightly spray an 8-inch baking dish with cooking spray and set aside.

In a bowl, mix together peaches, lemon juice, and arrowroot powder.

In a medium bowl, mix oats, cinnamon, vanilla, coconut oil, maple syrup, almond flour, pecans, and sea salt.

Transfer the peaches into the baking dish. Spread the oat mixture on top of the peaches evenly and press down using the back of the spoon.

Bake in preheated oven for 30 minutes.

Serve and enjoy.

Nutritional Data: 252 calories | 40.56g carbs | 12.26g fat | 3.13g protein | 81mg sodium

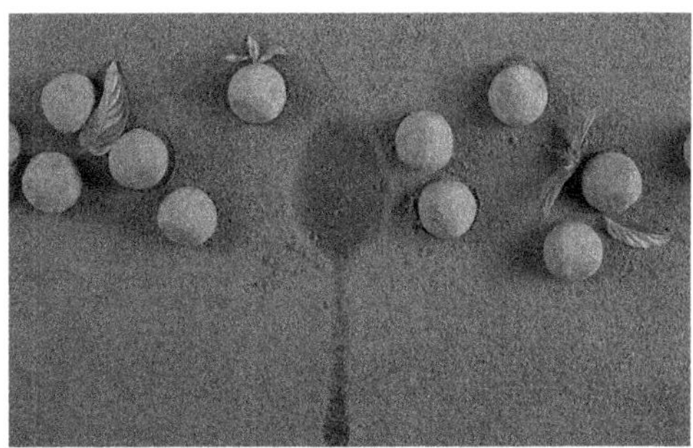

Preparation Time: 10 minutes
Cooking Time: 5 minutes
Serves: 20
Ingredients:

- 1 avocado, flesh scooped out
- 2 tbsp unsweetened cocoa powder
- 1 cup dark chocolate chips
- Sea salt

Directions:

Add chocolate chips into a microwave-safe bowl and microwave for 30 seconds or until chocolate is melted. Remove from microwave and stir until chocolate is smooth.

Add avocado, melted chocolate, and sea salt into a food processor and process until well combined.

Transfer avocado mixture into a bowl and place in refrigerator for 30 minutes or until firm.

Remove the avocado mixture from the refrigerator.

Add cocoa powder into a shallow bowl.

Make a 1-inch ball from the avocado mixture and roll in cocoa powder until coated. Place prepared balls onto a parchment-lined plate.

Store in refrigerator for 30 minutes.

Serve and enjoy.

Nutritional Data: 61 calories | 6.61g carbs | 3.88g fat | 0.66g protein | 38mg sodium

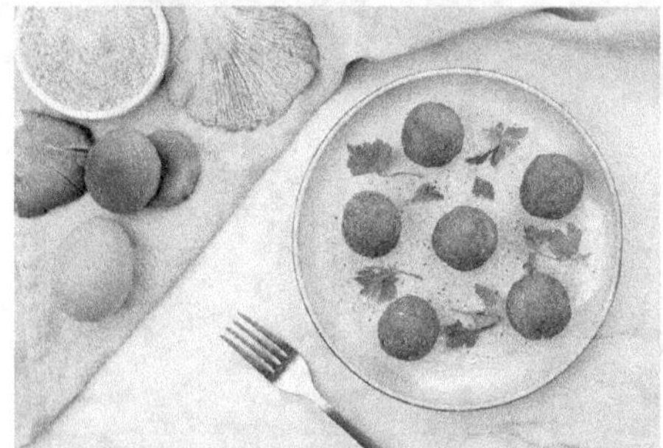

Preparation Time: 10 minutes
Cooking Time: 10 minutes
Serves: 28 balls
Ingredients:

- ½ cup carrots, chopped
- ½ tbsp maple syrup
- 1 tsp vanilla
- 3 tbsp peanut butter
- ¼ tsp ginger powder
- ½ tsp nutmeg
- ½ tsp cinnamon
- ½ cup oats
- 2 tbsp desiccated coconut
- ½ cup pecans
- ¼ cup dates, pitted

Directions:

Add dates and carrots into a food processor and process for 1 minute or until dates and carrots are cut into small pieces.

Add maple syrup, vanilla, peanut butter, ginger powder, nutmeg, cinnamon, oats, desiccated coconut, and pecans to the food processor and process until sticky dough forms.

Make equal shapes of balls from the mixture and place onto a plate.

Serve immediately and enjoy.

Nutritional Data: 28 calories | 3.31g carbs | 1.73g fat | 0.64g protein | 28mg sodium

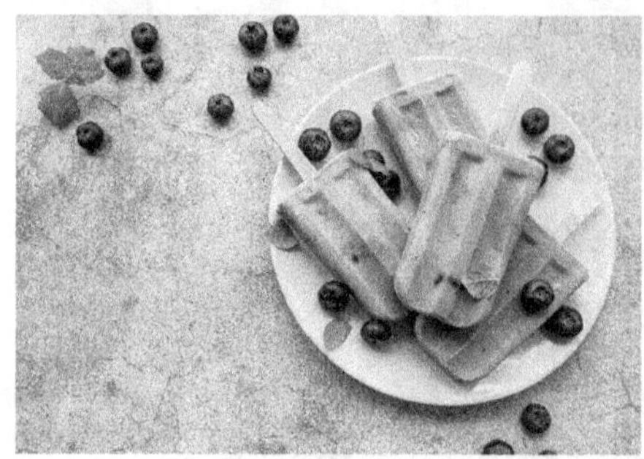

Preparation Time: 5 minutes
Cooking Time: 5 minutes
Serves: 10
Ingredients:

- 3 cups blueberries
- 14.5 oz full-fat coconut milk
- 2 tbsp maple syrup

Directions:

Add blueberries, coconut milk, and maple syrup into blender and blend until smooth.

Pour the blended mixture into popsicle mold and place it in the freezer overnight.

Serve and enjoy

Nutritional Data: 173 calories | 21.9g carbs | 10.06g fat | 1.44g protein | 9mg sodium

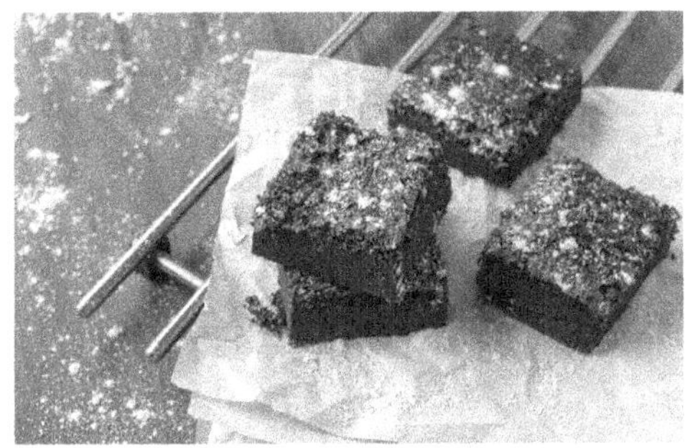

Preparation Time: 10 minutes
Cooking Time: 30 minutes
Serves: 9
Ingredients:

- 5 eggs
- ½ cup coconut flour
- ½ tsp baking soda
- 2 tbsp water
- 1/3 cup coconut oil, melted
- ½ cup honey
- ½ cup unsweetened cocoa powder
- 1/8 tsp sea salt

Directions:

Preheat oven to 350°F.

Line 8x8-inch baking dish with parchment paper and set aside.

In a medium bowl, mix together coconut flour, baking soda, cocoa powder, and sea salt.

In a mixing bowl, whisk together eggs, water, melted oil, and honey.

Slowly add the coconut flour mixture to the egg mixture and mix until well combined.

Pour batter into the prepared baking dish and bake in preheated oven for 30 minutes. Remove from oven and allow to cool completely.

Slice and serve.

Nutritional Data: 211 calories | 19.36g carbs | 14g fat | 6g protein | 177mg sodium

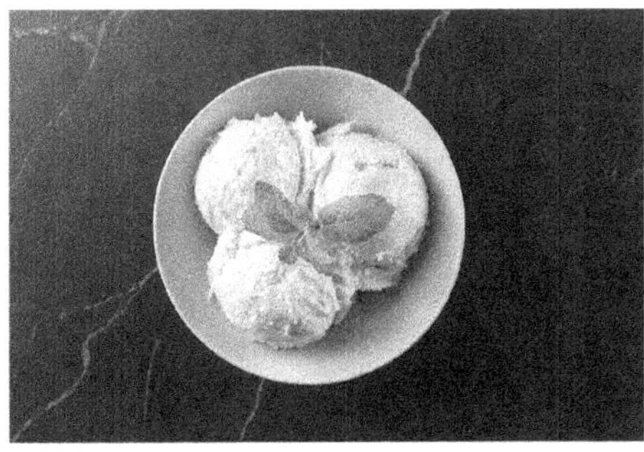

Preparation Time: 5 minutes
Cooking Time: 30 minutes
Serves: 6
Ingredients:

- 1 tbsp matcha green tea powder
- 29-oz can full-fat coconut milk
- ½ cup maple syrup

Directions:

Add matcha green tea powder, coconut milk, and maple syrup into blender and blend until combined.

Pour blended mixture into air-tight container and place in the freezer for 2 hours.

Add green tea ice cream base into your ice cream maker and churn according to your ice cream maker instructions, for about 30–40 minutes or until the ice cream is thick.

Serve immediately and enjoy

Nutritional Data: 383 calories | 25.19g carbs | 32.68g fat | 3.15g protein | 24mg sodium

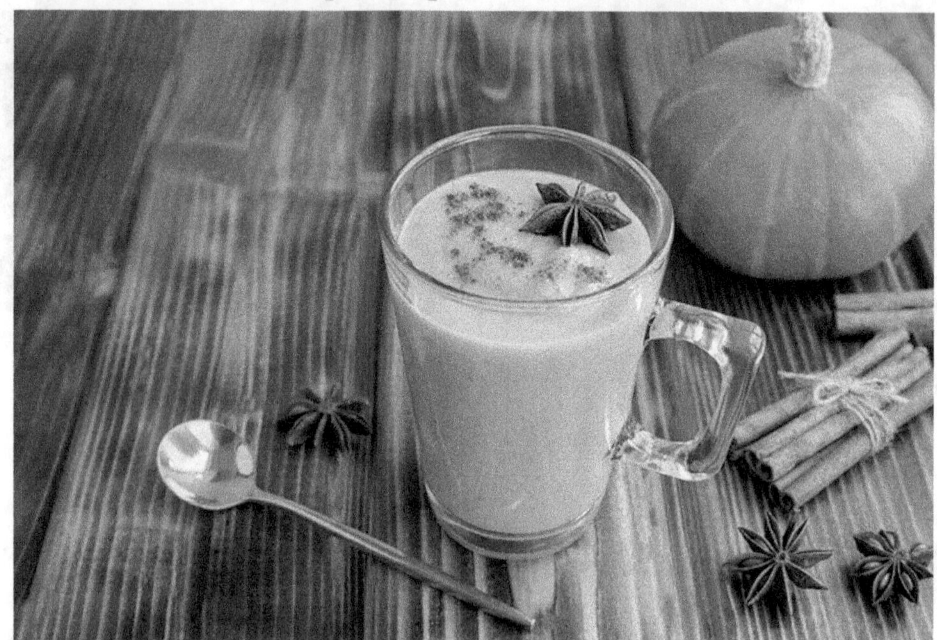

Preparation Time: 5 minutes
Cooking Time: 5 minutes
Serves: 2
Ingredients:

- 1 cup pumpkin puree
- ¼ cup strong coffee
- 1 tbsp maple syrup
- 1 banana
- ½ tsp pumpkin spice
- 2 cups unsweetened almond milk
- 1 cup ice cubes

Directions:

Add pumpkin puree and remaining ingredients into blender and blend until smooth and creamy.

Serve immediately and enjoy.

Nutritional Data: 682 calories | 66.35g carbs | 40.58g fat | 21.92g protein | 356mg sodium

Partnered with an anti-inflammatory diet, planning and cooking DASH meals for a month requires insightful ingredient selection that supports heart health and lowers inflammation. This 800-word guide below will help you compile a complete meal plan for the initial 30 days as per the DASH diet.

The DASH diet is a low-salt diet that is rich in potassium, calcium, and magnesium. It is also high in lean protein, fiber, and healthy fats. For an anti-inflammatory diet, it favors foods high in antioxidants, omega-3 fatty acids, and polyphenols. The food included in this diet plan will help reduce inflammation in the body.

Understand the Guidelines

The following are the food groups required for a DASH meal plan:

- **Vegetables and fruits:** 5 servings of vegetables and 4–5 servings of fruit per day. Eat a rainbow: more color, more nutrients. Green veggies, especially leafy greens and avocados, are great anti-inflammatory foods.
- **Lean proteins:** 1–2 servings of lean meats per day. Eat two servings of fish per week, especially fatty fish like salmon and mackerel.
- **Dairy:** 2–3 servings per day. In addition to unsalted dairy products, tofu and soy products should be consumed.
- **Nuts, seeds, and legumes:** 4–5 servings per week.
- **Whole Grains:** 90–225 grams of whole-wheat bread; 30–60 grams of brown rice, pasta, or crackers; 20–50 grams of dry oatmeal, quinoa, or whole-wheat cold cereal.
- **Fats, nuts, and seeds:** Up to 4–5 servings per week. Choose foods that are high in omega-3 fatty acids and antioxidants, and that have anti-inflammatory properties.
- **Sugar:** No more than 5 servings per week.

Planning Your Meals

Weekly Meal Planning

Think about setting up a meal rotation so that your diet stays interesting:

- **Week 1:** Introduce a wide range of whole grains and legumes. Try lots of different salad mixes, such as quinoa bean salad or a lentil-and-veggie stir-fry.
- **Week 2:** Introduce more seafood and start experimenting with fish cooked in different ways, for example grilled mackerel or baked salmon.
- **Week 3:** Increase the amount of raw veggies and fruits in your diet. Smoothies are a great, quick and easy way to pull this off.

- ➢ **Week 4:** Bring everything together from the previous weeks and consider including some low-fat dairy alternatives like almond or soy milk.

Daily Meal Planning

- ➢ **Eating plan:** Three main meals and two snacks should be consumed throughout the day. Here is an example of a day of meals:
- ➢ **Breakfast:** Whole-grain cereal and low-fat milk. Top with berries.
- ➢ **Mid-morning snack:** A small handful of almonds, mixed nuts, or a mixed fruit pack of dairy-free yogurt.
- ➢ **Lunch:** Wrap with lettuce, chicken, cold meats, or grilled vegetables (i.e., leftover from dinner), avocado, and a drizzle of olive oil (1/2–1 tsp OR 2–3 tsp fat-free salad dressing). Possible to add a large handful of baby spinach or other leafy greens.
- ➢ **Afternoon snack:** A few carrots and celery sticks with hummus or yogurt avocado dip.
- ➢ **Dinner:** Baked fish with quinoa or brown rice and steamed broccoli.

Preparing Your Ingredients

- ➢ **Batch cooking:** You may cook a week's worth of whole grains and legumes at the beginning of the week. This could be rice, quinoa, lentils, chickpeas, or black beans. You may also batch cook from meats. For example, grilling or baking all your fish one day so that you can quickly reheat it throughout the week.
- ➢ **Chopping vegetables:** Spend 30 minutes on the weekend cutting up veggies for the next two days and store them in airtight containers in the fridge. This way, you'll either throw them into a salad or quickly stir-fry them.
- ➢ **Portioning your snacks:** Make proffered nuts, seeds, cut fruit, and veggies at the beginning of the week for various portions of snacks and an easy snack out the door.

Execution and Adjustment

Stick to the meal plan but be flexible and willing to tweak it according to the produce available. Also, take into account your schedule. If a certain meal doesn't keep you full, tweak the portion or ingredients to serve your purpose.

Day 1
- Breakfast: Turmeric Oatmeal
- Lunch: Salmon Salad
- Dinner: Grilled Salmon with Asparagus

Day 2
- Breakfast: Chia Seed Pudding
- Lunch: Quinoa Salad
- Dinner: Vegetarian Chili

Day 3
- Breakfast: Avocado Toast
- Lunch: Tuna Lettuce Wraps
- Dinner: Lemon Herb Chicken

Day 4
- Breakfast: Smoothie Bowl
- Lunch: Turkey-and-Avocado Wrap
- Dinner: Stuffed Bell Peppers

Day 5
- Breakfast: Sweet Potato Hash
- Lunch: Vegetable Stir-Fry
- Dinner: Cauliflower Rice Stir-Fry

Day 6
- Breakfast: Quinoa Breakfast Bowl
- Lunch: Sweet Potato-and-Black Bean Bowl
- Dinner: Shrimp-and-Vegetable Skewers

Day 7
- Breakfast: Egg-and-Veggie Muffins
- Lunch: Mediterranean Chickpea Salad
- Dinner: Turkey Meatballs with Zoodles

Day 8
- Breakfast: Greek Yogurt Parfait
- Lunch: Egg Salad Lettuce Cups
- Dinner: Baked Cod with Roasted Vegetables

Day 9
- Breakfast: Tofu Scramble
- Lunch: Cauliflower Rice Bowl
- Dinner: Quinoa-Stuffed Acorn Squash

Day 10
- Breakfast: Coconut Flour Pancakes
- Lunch: Chicken-and-Vegetable Soup

Day 12
- Breakfast: Green Smoothie
- Lunch: Vegetable Stir-Fry
- Dinner: Zucchini Noodles with Pesto and Cherry Tomatoes

Day 13
- Breakfast: Almond Butter Banana Toast
- Lunch: Lentil Salad
- Dinner: Eggplant Parmesan

Day 14
- Breakfast: Berry Quinoa Breakfast Bake
- Lunch: Stuffed Bell Peppers
- Dinner: Cabbage Rolls

Day 15
- Breakfast: Cottage Cheese Bowl
- Lunch: Greek Yogurt Chicken Salad
- Dinner: Butternut Squash-and-Kale Salad

Day 16
- Breakfast: Egg-and-Veggie Stir-Fry
- Lunch: Sardine Salad Sandwich
- Dinner: Sesame Ginger Tofu Stir-Fry

Day 17
- Breakfast: Buckwheat Porridge
- Lunch: Spinach-and-Strawberry Salad
- Dinner: Mushroom-and-Spinach Risotto

Day 18
- Breakfast: Almond Flour Waffles
- Lunch: Shrimp-and-Avocado Salad
- Dinner: Baked Chicken with Brussels Sprouts

Day 19
- Breakfast: Mango Coconut Chia Pudding
- Lunch: Cabbage-and-Apple Slaw
- Dinner: Cauliflower Steak with Chimichurri Sauce

Day 20
- Breakfast: Sardine Toast
- Lunch: Butternut Squash Soup

- Dinner: Lentil-and-Sweet Potato Curry

Day 11
- Breakfast: Salmon-and-Avocado Wrap
- Lunch: Zucchini Noodles with Pesto
- Dinner:Spinach-and-Feta-Stuffed Chicken

Day 22
- Breakfast: Spinach-and-Mushroom Omelet
- Lunch: Caprese Salad
- Dinner: Stuffed Portobello Mushrooms

Day 23
- Breakfast: Pumpkin Smoothie
- Lunch: Eggplant-and-Chickpea Tagine
- Dinner: Pumpkin-and-Lentil Soup

Day 24
- Breakfast: Tomato Basil Avocado Toast
- Lunch: Tofu-and-Vegetable Stir-Fry
- Dinner: Coconut-Curry Chicken Skewers

Day 25
- Breakfast: Almond Butter Protein Balls
- Lunch: Cucumber-and-Avocado Soup
- Dinner: Roasted Vegetable-and-Chickpea Bowl

Day 26
- Breakfast: Turmeric Oatmeal
- Lunch: Lemon Herb Chicken Salad
- Dinner: Grilled Salmon with Asparagus

- Dinner: Vegetable-and-Bean Soup

Day 21
- Breakfast: Cinnamon Apple Oatmeal
- Lunch: Turkey-and-Vegetable Skewers
- Dinner: Salmon Cakes

Day 27
- Breakfast: Chia Seed Pudding
- Lunch: Salmon Salad
- Dinner: Vegetarian Chili

Day 28
- Breakfast: Avocado Toast
- Lunch: Quinoa Salad
- Dinner: Lemon Herb Chicken

Day 29
- Breakfast: Smoothie Bowl
- Lunch: Tuna Lettuce Wraps
- Dinner: Stuffed Bell Peppers

Day 30
- Breakfast: Sweet Potato Hash
- Lunch: Turkey-and-Avocado Wrap
- Dinner: Cauliflower Rice Stir-Fry

Eating out and staying on an anti-inflammatory diet can be very tough, but with a few tricks up your sleeve, you'll be able to make some delicious choices that don't derail your healthful priorities. Here are 10 tips to keep your anti-inflammatory diet plan on track when eating out.

- **Research the restaurant:** Look at the restaurant menu online before you go. A lot of restaurants have their menus online and they may even list allergen information or items that can be specially made diet-friendly.
- **Choose the right type of restaurant:** Stick with restaurants that are known for fresh, whole foods. Mediterranean, Japanese, and vegetarian restaurants generally have a variety of anti-inflammatory options.
- **Tell your server about your diet:** Ask your server or the chef about substitutions or how dishes are prepared. It's your right as a paying customer to have your food made how you want it.
- **Stay away from processed foods:** Fried, breaded, crispy, and other similar terms are telltale signs that a dish is high in unhealthy fats and processed ingredients. Look for dishes that are grilled, baked, or steamed, and order those instead.
- **Don't drown your dish in sugary dressings and unhealthy sauces:** Often, dressings and sauces are the most calorie-dense part of a dish. Ordering your dressings and sauces on the side ensures that you are in control of how much you use.
- **Vegetable load:** Ask for extra servings of vegetables and opt to find dishes where vegetables take center stage. That way, you'll be sure you are consuming enough antioxidants and fiber to reduce inflammation in your body.
- **Go for whole grain:** Whole-grain bread, rice, pasta, or anything of the sort are always better choices when available. The chances that whole grains will cause an inflammation reaction after eating are significantly lower than with the refined kind.
- **Lean protein:** Chicken, fish, or legumes are the way to go when picking a protein source. Fish, particularly fatty fish, is rich in omega-3 fatty acids which are known anti-inflammatory agents.
- **Stay hydrated:** Choose water, or herbal tea, but avoid sugar-sweetened beverages and alcohol which tend to start the inflammation process.

By adhering to these strategies, you can navigate the challenges of dining out while following an anti-inflammatory diet, ensuring that your meal not only satisfies your palate but also supports your health.

Conclusion

The anti-inflammatory diet is a relevant concept to the existing paradigm of health. Various health issues are linked to chronic inflammation: heart diseases, metabolism disorders such as type-2 diabetes, autoimmune conditions, arthritis, and several types of cancer. The diet addresses these issues by making sure that you have more opportunities to eat more whole, nutrient-dense foods while encountering fewer processed foods and bad fats. A nutrient-dense diet rich in multifunctional nutrients but low in processed foods and bad fats creates a nutritional environment that can alleviate inflammation and support health outcomes.

One of the benefits of following an anti-inflammatory diet is that it changes your eating habits, adding healthy whole foods, including a variety of fruits, vegetables, whole grains, legumes, nuts, seeds, and healthy fats such as those from fatty fish, olive oil, and avocados. These natural ingredients are packed with vitamins, minerals, fiber, and phytonutrients that work together to fight inflammation and strengthen the body's immune system—for example, the antioxidants abundant in fruits and vegetables, such as vitamin C, vitamin E, and beta carotene. They play an important role in combating stress and reducing inflammatory reactions in the body.

Another aspect of the anti-inflammatory diet is incorporating omega-3 acids from sources like fatty fish (salmon, sardines, mackerel) or plant-based options (flaxseeds, chia seeds, walnuts). Omega-3s are well-known for their inflammatory properties which help reduce inflammation markers while promoting heart health and brain function. Including these fats in your diet regularly can lead to improvements in managing inflammation and preventing diseases. Also, following an anti-inflammatory diet involves reducing intake of processed foods, added sugars, unhealthy fats, and refined grains. These types of foods have been linked to triggering responses and causing metabolic issues. By cutting back on these triggers you not only reduce inflammation but also lower insulin resistance, thus decreasing the risk of developing chronic conditions associated with long-term inflammation.

Finally, one other important principle of the anti-inflammatory diet is proper sources of protein. The preferable types of protein foods are plant-based protein foods (legumes, tofu and tempeh, quinoa), and lean-on animal sources of protein (poultry and fish). You should strive to include plant-based proteins provided in your daily ration to get crucial amino acids that promote optimal health. They have exclusive properties; for example, due to reduced consumption of rare protein sources like red meat, you will feel more confident about lean ones, which help to keep a metabolic profile healthful as well as maintain the body in an anti-inflammatory state, fitting contemporary nutritional research standards. Another assumption within the anti-inflammatory diet in addition to dietary shifts is the use of anti-inflammatory herbs and spices. Among the recommended are turmeric, ginger, garlic, cinnamon, and rosemary due to their active anti-inflammatory bioactive compounds. Therefore, introducing these kinds of herbs and spices into the diet can potentiate it through a curative perspective. For instance, curcumin is the most active compound of turmeric, and numerous studies were conducted to understand its anti-inflammatory properties. Hence, the anti-inflammatory diet may be modified by different components and approaches.

There is more than the dietary approach to beat inflammation in this diet; physical activity, lifestyle, and mindset also play a huge role in the management of inflammation. A healthy lifestyle not only encourages more physical exercise, which is anti-inflammatory in many but not all immune system compartments, but it also increases circulation. Better blood flow stimulates the sympathetic nervous system. Stress management through practices like meditation, yoga, or deep breathing techniques can decrease cortisol levels which will result in an anti-inflammatory effect. One of the most important things that can play a role in regulating inflammation is sleep. Sleep deprivation is associated with increased pro-inflammatory cytokines and decreased immune function.

In general, the constructs of the anti-inflammatory diet look promising in defining pharmacological and multi-sectorial principles of the best integrative healthy-living formula. There are, however, caveats and several limitations. Individual responses to anti-inflammatory dietary interventions may be different due to genetic, metabolic, and comorbid profiles. Conversely, strict adherence to the anti-inflammatory diet recommendations can also be of high hazard for patients who do not belong to the Western culture, live in an unfavorable socio-economic status, or fit the behavioral phenotype specific to their needs.

So, the anti-inflammatory diet can be an incredibly potent tool in both preventing and potentially even reversing many of the factors that contribute to chronic diseases and, therefore, optimizing overall health. By ensuring that our bodies receive the nutrients they need while alleviating them from the burden of foods they struggle to process, the anti-inflammatory diet is a powerful way to support the body's most high-performing systems. And because it's not impossible to forego fast food, processed junk, and the occasional sweet treat for at least some of the time, anti-inflammatory diets can be beneficial to everyone. The evidence is clear: it's fundamental to the bigger health picture. Ending inflammation in the body can help keep us free from inflammation-related chronic diseases and promote a long health span full of energy!

Reference Page

Anti-inflammatory diet. (2024, February 20). Johns Hopkins Medicine. https://www.hopkinsmedicine.org/health/wellness-and-prevention/anti-inflammatory-diet

Chan Zuckerberg Initiative. (2022, November 30). *Causes of inflammation and how it affects health - CZI blog*. https://chanzuckerberg.com/blog/causes-symptoms-inflammation/

Fletcher, J. (2023, September 6). *Anti-inflammatory diet: What to know*. https://www.medicalnewstoday.com/articles/320233

Inhc, A. C. A. (2021, December 30). *What is the Anti-Inflammatory diet?* Verywell Fit. https://www.verywellfit.com/anti-inflammatory-diet-4649944

Lawler, M. (2023, February 24). *Anti-Inflammatory Diet: Diet: how it works, benefits, foods, and more*. EverydayHealth.com. https://www.everydayhealth.com/diet-nutrition/diet/anti-inflammatory-diet-benefits-food-list-tips/

Ld, L. W. M. R. (2023a, May 23). *Anti-Inflammatory foods to eat: A full list*. Healthline. https://www.healthline.com/nutrition/13-anti-inflammatory-foods

Ld, L. W. M. R. (2023b, May 23). *Anti-Inflammatory foods to eat: A full list*. Healthline. https://www.healthline.com/nutrition/13-anti-inflammatory-foods

Ld, S. S. M. R. (2022, April 13). *7-Day meal plan to Fight inflammation: Recipes and more*. Healthline. https://www.healthline.com/nutrition/7-day-meal-plan-to-fight-inflammation-recipes-and-more

Mph, T. C. (2023, May 5). *What is inflammation?* Health. https://www.health.com/inflammation-7480642

Nutritionist, K. T. –. (2024, March 20). *Top 10 anti-inflammatory foods*. Good Food. https://www.bbcgoodfood.com/howto/guide/top-10-anti-inflammatory-foods

RDN, J. J. M. (2024, January 9). 5 Anti-Inflammatory diets you should Try. *Forbes Health*. https://www.forbes.com/health/nutrition/diet/anti-inflammatory-diets-to-try/

Spritzler, F. (2023, October 12). *What is an Anti-Inflammatory Diet and How to Follow it*. Healthline. https://www.healthline.com/nutrition/anti-inflammatory-diet-101#foods-to-eat

What is Acute Inflammation? CUSABIO. (n.d.). CUSABIO. https://www.cusabio.com/Immunology/Acute-Inflammation.html

www.ingramcontent.com/pod-product-compliance
Lightning Source LLC
Chambersburg PA
CBHW081554250726
48653CB00009B/3430